Wakefield Press

Radiance in Pain and Resilience

Dr Samah Jabr, a consultant psychiatrist practicing in Palestine, serving communities in East Jerusalem and the West Bank, is Head of the Mental Health Unit within the Palestinian Ministry of Health. She is an Associate Clinical Professor of Psychiatry and Behavioral Sciences at George Washington University in Washington DC. Dr Jabr is a trainer and supervisor with a special focus on Cognitive Behavioral Therapy (CBT), mhGAP, and the Istanbul Protocol for the documentation of torture. She frequently consults on program development for international organizations. Her key interests include the rights of prisoners, suicide prevention, and historical trauma.

In addition to her clinical work, Dr Jabr has dedicated over two decades to advocating on behalf of the mental healthcare of the Palestinian people, focusing on victims of torture and trauma. She is the author of several books, including *Behind the Frontlines: Chronicles of a Palestinian Psychiatrist Psychotherapist under Occupation*, *Sumud: Resisting Oppression*, *Sumud in Times of Genocide*, and *The Time of Genocide: Bearing Witness to a Year in Palestine*; many of these have been published in multiple languages. Dr Jabr integrates her medical expertise with her activism, often addressing the psychological impact of occupation, historical trauma, and war. She is a founding member of the Palestine Global Mental Health Network, and a prolific speaker on liberation psychology and the ethical responsibilities of mental health professionals in conflict zones.

'A brave and beautiful book, an essential elixir of truth, a cry to and from the heart. It will hurt, it will educate, and it will inspire.'

—Gabor Maté MD

By the same author

Behind the Frontlines: Chronicles of a Palestinian Psychiatrist Psychotherapist under Occupation
(appeared in French, Italian and Spanish)

Sumud: Resisting Oppression
(appeared in Italian)

Sumud in Times of Genocide
(appeared in Portuguese)

The Time of Genocide: Bearing Witness to a Year in Palestine
(appeared in Italian)

Radiance in Pain and Resilience

The Global Reverberation of Palestinian Historical Trauma

Samah Jabr

Foreword by Gabor Maté

Wakefield Press

Wakefield Press
16 Rose Street
Mile End
South Australia 5031
www.wakefieldpress.com.au

First published 2025

Edited by Julia Beaven, Wakefield Press
Text designed and typeset by Jesse Pollard, Wakefield Press

ISBN 978 1 92304 292 6

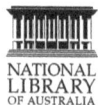

A catalogue record for this
book is available from the
National Library of Australia

To the steadfast people of Palestine,

Your resilience in the face of relentless adversity is the foundation of this work.

To the martyrs and those who mourn them, to the rescue teams who pull children from beneath the rubble, to the healthcare workers, doctors and journalists who risk everything to restore dignity to the dehumanized, and to the activists and freedom fighters—both in Palestine and beyond—your courage and sacrifice shape the conscience of the world.

To all who carry Palestine in their hearts, proving that this struggle is not bound by geography or identity, may your stories of endurance and defiance continue to inspire.

To the fragmented land, the dispossessed people, and those whose bodies have been broken but whose spirits remain whole—I write with the hope that, together, we will reclaim what is ours.

My deepest gratitude to our friends at the Shifa Project, whose solidarity strengthens our path, to the publishing team, and to my dedicated editor, Julia Beaven, for her thoughtful guidance. I am especially grateful to a dear brother in spirit, Ziyad Serhan, for his unwavering support, and above all, to my friend and colleague, Zaynab Hinnawi, whose companionship and commitment mean more than words can express.

Samah Jabr

Contents

Mental Health Under Occupation

Occupation is a Mental Health Issue

About Resistance and Resilience

About Solidarity

Epilogue

Final Words

Foreword

Gabor Maté MD, Author of *The Myth of Normal: Trauma, Illness and Healing in a Toxic Culture*

How to approach a book that breaks your heart yet compels you not to avert your eyes, that demands you to bear witness to one of the great tragedies of our current moment and of the past century? My answer is: with reverence, with a willingness to access our capacity to learn, to mourn, to be outraged, and to be stirred to action.

As these words are penned, there is a temporary ceasefire in Gaza that is allowing a grief-stricken, devastated and decimated population to return to the rubble and ruins of their homes, hospitals, schools, graveyards, even as their compatriots in the West Bank are under relentless assault by rampaging settlers and the IDF. Who knows when this fragile peace, if we can call it so, will be shattered once again—as it likely will be before this book goes to print. That is the context from which this volume, this report from the front lines of health under siege, emanates, this cri-de-coeur of a psychiatrist whose birth, childhood, entire life, training and career have been shadowed by her people's ongoing trauma—a trauma, as Dr Samah Jabr points out, "not limited to a single catastrophic event, but continues over an extended period of time." One that "derails the population from its natural developmental course—resulting in a legacy of physical, psychological, social, and economic discontinuities that are transmitted intergenerationally and persist."

As Head of Mental Health in occupied Palestine, Dr Jabr understands better than most Western medical colleagues that health, physical and mental—not that the two can be split—is a bio-psycho-social phenomenon. That is, the functioning of people's minds and brains cannot be separated from the experience of their bodies in a cultural context, situated in historical circumstances. And the historical circumstances of the Palestinian people have been characterized by violence directed against them for nearly eight decades now—or if we add, as we should, the British imperial occupation under which they languished prior to the establishment of the State of Israel—for over a century. "Political violence interacts with the individual bio-psychosocial vulnerabilities to provoke illness," she writes. Israeli state violence can be, and often is, directly physical, as in killings, maiming, beatings, torture, destruction of homes. I have personally worked with Palestinian torture victims, witnessed the home destructions, seen the arbitrary indignities visited upon ordinary people, but even I was struck by the case histories Dr Samah Jabr reports—such as that of an elderly man who presented with suicidal ideation after having been coerced to personally dismantle the home he had built with his own hands 20 years earlier!

The violence is also inflicted in psychological ways such as the humiliation of parents in front of their children, the denial of Palestinian history, the forced participation in rituals that honor the occupier, the separation of families, the uncertainty and arbitrary issuance or denial of passes allowing access to services, relatives and health care. And in myriad other ways that a truly ingenious colonial system can devise to break the will, self-esteem, unity, mental resilience and capacity to resist of an oppressed population.

As a psychotherapist, Dr Jabr must help alleviate in individuals the impacts of trauma imposed on a whole nation. "I try to help people make sense of their painful experiences by creating an explanatory, validating narrative that gathers the complexity of their situation and negotiates their conflict with oppressive powers, rather than labeling them with a diagnostic code," she writes.

Lest anyone fall for the canard that history and conflict began on October 7, 2023, this book also includes dispatches written many years earlier. The book, based on articles and talks by the author, is organized around themes such as the experience of the family under occupation—predictably, one of increasing dislocation and alienation and transgenerational trauma transmission or, say, mental health under occupation—a subject that renders risible labels such as "post-traumatic stress disorder." As I have observed in my visits to the Occupied Territories, and as Dr Jabr amply documents, there is no "post" in Palestine. The trauma is ever-present, relentless, and is becoming more ominous and relentless each year.

Abundantly illustrated by clinical case histories—each one as illuminating as heartrending—this book is also a forthright and courageous pollical statement. It does not spare the Palestinian enablers of the occupation, their opportunism or corruption. Nor does it ignore the pernicious influence of the international health organizations whose "help" either indirectly, if unwittingly, supports the agenda of occupation or who—most egregiously, the American Psychiatric Association—focus their empathy only on the Israeli victims of spasmodic Palestinian violence while utterly ignoring and even justifying the long-term history and current practices of the Zionist state, practices that prominent Jewish Israeli scholars of genocide (such as Profs Omer Bartov and Raz Segal) have called genocidal. It is a project of which the Western media have been shameless accomplices, helping to perpetuate what Dr Jabr aptly calls "the assassination of Palestinian memory." Or, we might add, the assassination of any memory of Palestine in the Western mind.

As to the future? Current UN estimates say that that 92% of Gazan residences have been destroyed or significantly damaged, as has two thirds of the infrastructure, including health-care facilities, hospitals, schools, and so on. The rubble, mixed with toxic chemicals and explosive ordnance, will take at least a decade and a half to clear—that is, if such work is permitted by the occupier. And only if the work of clearing and reconstruction is not further impeded by ongoing military action, and by the ethnic cleansing implicit in the Zionist idea and now openly embraced by segments of the Israeli leadership and actively or passively tolerated by much of the Israeli public.

Yet this book ends with hope—or, better, with faith. Faith in humanity and, specifically, in the spirit of the Palestinian people. "The Palestinian narrative is one fraught with displacement, dispossession, and cultural distortion interwoven with threads of struggle and resilience," Dr Jabr reminds us. The Palestinian word *sumud*, for which resilience is itself a paltry translation, involves "not accepting the status quo . . . Sumud means maintaining optimism, moral and social solidarity while dealing with grim realities and oppressive structure. [It is] that painful position of searching for our lost freedom with the hope that we will find it one day."

As an infant survivor of the Nazi genocide, I used to believe in the dream of Jewish redemption Zionism represented. I have long ago seen what a nightmare the realization of that dream has imposed on the Palestinians, and what a catastrophe it has been and even more, will be, for the Jewish people as well. Anyone who cares about human dignity and freedom and health, and especially anyone who wants to awaken to present realities, will find this brave and beautiful book an essential elixir of truth, a cry to and from the heart. It will hurt, it will educate, and it will inspire.

Gabor Maté MD, 2025

Foreword

Elizabeth Berger MD, Associate Clinical Professor of Psychiatry and Behavioral Sciences, George Washington University School of Medicine and Health Sciences, Washington, DC,

It is an honor, a joy, and a responsibility to welcome this book and to introduce Dr Samah Jabr to a wide public audience. The moment could hardly be more urgent.

Few today can ignore indications of the ongoing slaughter of thousands of innocent civilians in Palestine as well as the needless deaths of many others in the Middle East; few today are confident in grasping the meaning of this human catastrophe. As witnesses, we are perplexed and exhausted. A morally sound, informed, and coherent global response is desperately needed. But what response? How can we understand these appalling losses and what we can do about them?

The doctor is here.

This volume collects in one place dozens of brilliant essays on Palestine—for the most part previously published in English over the past decade for a general audience. The essays are brief, lyrical, fascinating, and accessible. Each addresses a facet of the Palestinian situation through the eyes of one woman who is simultaneously a practicing psychiatrist, international consultant, research scholar, and public intellectual. Dr Samah is currently the Head of the Mental Health Unit within the Palestinian Ministry of Health in Ramallah, Palestine, and responsible for setting the course of mental health care in the West Bank. Her work "away from her desk" is tireless—writing, speaking, and teaching on behalf of the people of Palestine and in defense of human rights everywhere.

The beauty of bringing together these various essays lies in its comprehensive human vision, expressed with clarity, compassion, and ferocious dedication to the ideal of justice. This vision speaks above all to the deep need for dignity as a crucial element of wellbeing and the relevance of the socio-political context to any individual's capacity to experience wellbeing. Acknowledging the centrality of freedom, and the universal struggle for freedom, is thus inseparable from the doctor's archaic duty to address suffering. The "medical model" here is not separated from a profound meditation on the needs of the human spirit, but integrated within it.

Dr Samah and I have been friends and colleagues for many years, working together on various clinical and educational projects in Palestine as well as co-authoring academic journal articles and book chapters written for a professional audience. Dr Samah has been a prime force in the development of the mental health advocacy organization, the Palestine-Global Mental Health Network, and its 14 supportive solidarity networks established in a variety of countries internationally. My own work with Dr Samah, and the work of our wonderful and ever-growing legion of comrades everywhere, has given rise to deep friendships and a renewed faith in human goodness.

This volume, dear reader, invites us to understand more fully the concrete experience of the people of Palestine and to situate its immediate horrors in historical perspective. At the same time, this book provides a steadfast point of view, illuminating the realities of Palestine but speaking with wisdom and a measure of hope to the needs of human beings everywhere. This is a gift to all of us.

Let the doctor speak for herself.

Elizabeth Berger MD, 2024

Introduction

Therapy, Awareness and Critical Consciousness

Originally published in *Our Vision For Liberation: Engaged Palestinian Leaders & Intellectuals Speak Out*, Ramzy Baroud and Ilan Pappe, November 2021

I came to life with an injury and pain. I weighed 5300 grams at birth, which took place through an ordinary vaginal delivery. However, because of my large size, the delivery was so difficult that, in order to save my life and that of my mother, the doctors had to break my clavicle. This caused permanent injury to the underlying left brachial plexus—the nerves connected to my supposedly dominant arm. For years afterwards my parents carried me, as they went on foot from Shufat to the French Hill so I could receive physiotherapy sessions at an Israeli medical center. I continued that treatment well into the time that I developed the capacity to remember what I experienced.

I remember Riva, the practitioner who was taking care of me—an Israeli woman who I now recognize as a religious Jew, on the basis of her appearance. I remember the yellow ladders I had to climb to strengthen my atrophying arm. This was a difficult exercise and I undertook it only to receive the chocolate I earned when I finished my training for the day. I also remember very well how exhausting this trip was for my parents, who did not have a car or speak Hebrew, and were apprehensive about the dominating Israeli presence in the center. These trips were especially hard on my mother, who would return home tired and sunburnt after the morning's journey; I remember her making a yoghurt-based emulsion to ease the sun's effect on her face.

I had been the fourth girl in a row. My sisters were closer to one another in age; my mother had given birth to a stillborn baby boy just before me, and then had to cope with the difficult delivery and my injury. I highly suspect that she suffered from post-partum depression after my birth. I also know that I was given the name Samah, meaning forgiveness, to make up for the disappointment of a fourth baby girl.

In primary school, I was overweight and myopic, with thick corrective eyeglasses. I was a "clumsy" child and therefore not a great physical play partner. When I joined play, I was often blamed for the team losing the game. The weakness in my arm and its limitation of movement caused me frequent injuries and led to the formation of multiple scars on my forehead and scalp. Perhaps this early experience as a bit of a misfit made me sensitive and empathic to other people who have difficulty integrating—such as classmates with learning disabilities and students who came from a difficult social background.

On the other hand, my subtle physical weaknesses gave me a strong motivation to develop my brain muscles. I was very good at playing with words and stood out as a popular and reliable colleague and friend. I was labeled "the advocate" by schoolmates who sought my help when in trouble, and who asked me to write letters on their behalf to the teachers and administration. Likewise, I was labeled an "argumentative troublemaker" by the adults, but still esteemed as a wise child. As one might have anticipated, I was punished several times for standing up for my rights and the rights of others in the face of strong and powerful adults.

My adolescence, during the collective experience of the First Intifada, accentuated these early childhood traits. I was aware of being viewed as part of a broken, dysfunctional, defective community, and this interaction between the personal and the collective accelerated my development of a sophisticated understanding of politics and power dynamics. I developed hypertrophic qualities of openness, authenticity and autonomy, to the point that my friend, Betsy Mayfield, used to tell me, "You are embracing the world with one arm." My mother used to warn me in a similar vein, "You can't hold a big watermelon under one arm and not expect it to fall down."

As a wise adolescent, aware of my parents' anxieties, societal prohibitions and political oppression, I was keen to calculate risks so as to avoid putting them, or myself, in danger. The courage, caution and critical thinking I developed during my adolescence have helped me walk the narrow alleys and to navigate a path to love and freedom through many subsequent dangers: the Israeli occupation, the oppression by Palestinian institutions, societal corruption, patriarchy and sexism and, as my world got bigger, I had to also deal with Western Islamophobia and complicity against my people. My adolescence equipped me for a long journey in the pursuit of well-being and liberty for myself, for my loved ones and for the injured Palestinian community.

I armed myself with studying and working hard in medicine, followed by specialization in psychiatry. Several theories of psychotherapy seemed appropriate for the mission of healing the traumatized individuals I encountered in clinical settings. Yet, I had to find "treatment" for the ill relationships caused among individuals, which weakened the cohesion of a community under military occupation. Collaboration with Israelis, pervasive distrust in ourselves, and a collective sense of inferiority and helplessness are just a few symptoms of an oppressed community. I found it equally important to maintain close observation of the direct experience of people. I learned to draw my conclusions from the ground up and to seek remedies for historical and collective trauma in promoting agency, self-direction and wellness within individuals, within community development, and through social and political action.

My work has been extremely varied. It has included policymaking and the development of national strategies, such as a national suicide prevention strategy and a national mental health response plan to COVID-19. It has also included extensive involvement in providing training and supervision for doctors and mental health workers, which contributes to building professional capacities and liberal and ethical attitudes in future mental health practice in Palestine. In addition, I have had a wide range of clinical experience with patients suffering from psychosis and other severe mental disorders; families with battered women in shelters, civil law prisoners, political prisoners, juvenile offenders and victims of trauma due to political violence and torture. In all of these groups, I see how political violence interacts with the individual bio-psychosocial vulnerabilities to provoke illness and impede recovery.

I also support the struggles of those I encounter outside the clinic—demoralized people oscillating between survival and surrender under oppression and enduring social ills, such as patriarchy, gender-based violence, corruption, nepotism, institutional hypocrisy and the subtle pernicious way of flattening and evacuating the values and belief systems of Palestinians and imposing false values on them by oppressive political powers.

The exaggerated celebrations of high school exams, while inhibiting and punishing any critical thinking in Palestinian universities and any freedom of expression on social media is an example of this falsification.

When people protested against the official assassination of Palestinian opposition activist Nizar Banat, official media diffused the situation, claiming that those people have an "external agenda" and that the women who participated in the demonstrations have no "honor" and their slogans "scratch the purity" of the Palestinian society. The mobile phones of the female participants were confiscated and their content was used as a subject to blackmail, silence and hypovisibilize them. Like Israel's agents who pose as Palestinians to assassinate activists in our markets and camps, Palestinian official security agents sneaked into opposition demonstrations wearing civilian clothes and started attacking the demonstrators with stones in order to break their bones; images that remind us of the behavior of soldiers following the orders of Yitzhak Rabin to break Palestinians' legs and arms. All of the above are Israeli tactics, copied by the Palestinian security system that does not only identify, but is also fascinated, with the aggressor.

Activism through writing, public speaking, mobilization and networking with friends, colleagues and comrades, and advocacy for social and political justice have become interventions to heal the social ills burdening the occupied Palestinian community. I engage in this work as a conscientious citizen, pressured by the heavy weight of crushing oppression, not as an external expert looking on from afar.

Like many other Palestinians, my life is characterized by the theft of both space and time. In Jerusalem, where space is shrinking for the Palestinian residents, neighbors can kill each other for a parking spot for their cars or for an empty space on the roof of their shared buildings. I am aware of these strangulating constraints, as I live through the resulting aggression of this reality on my skin. My personal survival strategy includes hyper-functioning and politically analyzing this reality, as I live on the crossroad of the two worlds of Jerusalem and the West Bank. I feel that the chronic lateness and deliberate slowness of bureaucracy and administration are yet other tools to suffocate the people of Palestine. Liberation will mean taking possession of our space and our time, and using them wisely, an issue that I struggle to explain to friends outside Palestine.

Generating and sharing Palestinian local knowledge with the world is another battlefield for me and other Palestinian scholars. Our special relationship with time and the lack of appropriate budget and personnel are just a few obstacles to generating mental health knowledge. Scholarly writing takes endless effort in footnoting, proofreading and formatting, and often requires authors or readers to pay to have the journal, or its articles, forwarded to colleagues. Conferences are expensive to attend, even when one is presenting at the conference.

While I rely on confident colleagues to help me co-author academic papers to transmit Palestinian local knowledge and expertise, I also try to simplify and explain relevant international academic knowledge to Palestinians. The abstruse lingo of much academic writing can be above the heads of many people who are involved in social and political change. Instead, I would rather spend my time rendering the sophisticated language of academia intelligibly and popularly. I prefer to draw applicable points and bring take-home messages to ordinary people who can benefit from them.

With my growing reputation and authority as a leading Palestinian and regional mental health professional, comes pressure to write ambiguous medico-legal reports that are dictated by powerful authorities and serve their specific interests—another challenge which eats into my physical and mental health. Working hard to earn my reputation and financial independence are my strategies to stand up to, and to resist, this kind of seduction and pressure.

I use my authority as a professional to advocate for an increase in staff and budget for mental health and to oppose stigma, ignorant myths, and discrimination against women, queer people and the most vulnerable in the community. I try to promote psychiatric treatment outside the psychiatric hospital and integrate mental health in primary health care and general hospitals.

I try to encourage contextualizing Palestinian psychological thinking, questioning the Western concept of PTSD, exploring important notions like "jihad", "shaheed", "sacrifice", "betrayal", "honor", "sumud", "resistance", "homeland", "solidarity"—and other influential concepts relevant to the Palestinian vision for liberation. I see the work of clarifying these concepts as a contribution to dismantling established and entrenched systems of injustice.

I have no illusions of omnipotence, but I will try to live long enough to leave behind a meaningful contribution in the liberation project of Palestine. I find that the liberation of the mind, through therapy, awareness and critical consciousness as fundamental to this project and this is the area where I can contribute the most.

This day marks 45 years of holding a weak and painful arm to my body, as well as a partially weak and painful representation of Palestine in my mind. My physical experience has taught me something about asymmetry, power imbalances and tilting. Nevertheless, I know how to get around the weakness in my arm whenever I wash my face, cut my steak, drive my car and give a big strong hug to my loved ones. I use this experiential knowledge and understanding to undertake counter-maneuvers during moments of weakened morale, and I continue to wrestle with power relations and fight for the liberation of occupied Palestine.

Gaza

In the Battle for Liberation, Gaza is Closer to Jerusalem than Ramallah

Originally published on *Middle East Monitor*, 12 May 2021

Ramadan has been a tense month in Jerusalem; it started with the Israelis forbidding Palestinian Jerusalemites from using the area at the Damascus Gate as a public space for social and cultural activities, in their effort to undermine the identity and significance of the place for the Palestinian community. Last year, the Israeli municipality of Jerusalem changed the area's name and erected a sign at the Damascus Gate reading in Hebrew "*Ma'Alot Hadar VaHadas*" (in English, "The Hadar and Hadas Steps"), in memory of the Israeli border police officers Hadar Cohen and Hadas Malka, who were killed in confrontations with Palestinians at the Damascus Gate in 2016 and 2017, respectively. But the Arabic name of Damascus Gate as it is known to Palestinians is Bab El-Amud, meaning "the Gate of the Column". This name makes reference to a black marble column 14 metres high which had been placed in the inner square of the door during the ancient Roman period. Distances from Jerusalem were measured from this column.

Over the past month, Palestinians have held daily sit-ins in increasing numbers at Bab El-Amud, in spite of the escalating attacks by occupation forces. The demonstrating Palestinians have endured beatings, tear gas and skunk water from Israeli soldiers, as well as attacks and threats to burn yet more Palestinians and their villages at the hands of extreme Israeli settler groups such as Lehava.

On 22 April, hundreds of far-right and anti-Palestinian activists took to the streets of Jerusalem's Old City, chanting "Death to the Arabs". *Haaretz* revealed that Israeli far-right organisations had used WhatsApp groups to call upon protesters to carry guns while posting instructions on how to avoid arrest. The *Haaretz* article quoted a comment in a group chat for far-right group La Familia events: "Burning Arabs today. Molotov cocktails are already in the trunk . . . the way I see it, an Arab dies today." During these events, we saw several videos of Israeli soldiers brutally beating and stepping on the heads of Palestinian protesters. After two weeks of daily confrontation, the Israeli police backed off in front of steadfast Palestinian youth.

Earlier this year, the Israeli Central Court of East Jerusalem decided to forcibly displace four families from the Sheikh Jarrah neighbourhood in favour of Israeli settlers who declared their intent to build a settlement of 200 residential units in the neighbourhood. After a long juridical process, the Israeli Supreme Court was due to issue a similar ruling on 10 May. Several other families in the same neighbourhood face the same predicament.

Those families whose homes are targeted by the Israelis today were originally refugees expelled from their homes during the 1948 Nakba. In 1956, these families were subsequently protected through a housing agreement with the Jordanian Ministry of Construction and Development and with the United Nations Relief and Works Agency (UNRWA). According to this agreement, the Jordanian government provided the land under Jordanian rule, UNRWA paid for the construction of 28 homes, and the residents paid a symbolic fee signifying that ownership was to be transferred to them in due course. The 1967 occupation of East Jerusalem interrupted this process.

The claim that these homes belong to Israeli settlers is based on a 1970 statement from the Israeli Department of Legal and Administrative Affairs, which permits Jewish Israelis to reclaim property lost in East Jerusalem in 1948. Meanwhile, the Absentees' Property Law of 1950 applies to non-Jewish Palestinians, including those who became citizens of the State of Israel but were not in their usual place of residence as defined by the law; this law prevents Palestinians from reclaiming the land from which they were expelled. According to international law, however, East Jerusalem, including the Sheikh Jarrah neighbourhood, is occupied land and it is unlawful under the Fourth Geneva Convention for an occupying power to transfer members of its own population into the territory it occupies. International humanitarian law prohibits the establishment of settlements, as these are a form of population transfer into occupied territory.

The families of Sheikh Jarrah and all Palestinians who are watching this happen are therefore experiencing déjà vu of the events of 1947—especially at this time of the year when we are about to commemorate the Nakba itself, the military actions that led to the expulsion of two-thirds of the Palestinian population from their homes. These thoughts of the Nakba engendered feelings of solidarity among many Palestinian Jerusalemites as well as activists from other areas of 1948 Palestine who had arrived to sit in support of the families of Sheikh Jarrah during the month of Ramadan, and who were also subjected to attacks by both soldiers and settlers.

On Monday, the 28th of Ramadan, Israeli forces launched a huge attack on Palestinian worshippers practicing Itikaf, a retreat into the mosque from daily life taking place during the last ten days of Ramadan. They injured hundreds in their effort to expel Muslim worshippers to prepare the area for the thousands of settlers who planned to march to Jerusalem's Old City, dancing with Israeli flags to celebrate the occupation of Jerusalem, which they call the unification of Jerusalem. We could see their euphoric dance and hear their genocidal chanting "their names to be deleted", in reference to the Palestinians—as they saw a fire at Al-Aqsa Mosque.

Palestinian Jerusalemites stand alone with only very local and grass-root organisations, lacking political leadership, in the face of growing Israeli brutality. Israel takes advantage of the ineffective official Palestinian leadership and the recent official surrender of four Arab regimes into a shameless normalisation process.

The war on Jerusalemites and their ethnic cleansing has been relentless through yet more subtle policies. The Israelis have imposed the Israeli curricula in the majority of Palestinian schools; the dropout rate in schools is 13 per cent. The vast majority of Jerusalemites live below the poverty line. Policies that aim to eliminate Palestinians have been effective in throwing many of us out of the borders of Jerusalem; the engineering plan for the city grants 100 annual construction permits for Palestinians while allowing 1500 for Jewish Israelis. Marriage to a non-Jerusalemite shatters families and breaks the household.

Palestinian Jerusalemites are citizens of nowhere—everywhere threatened, suspected, searched, accused, targeted with drugs and brainwashing for assimilation, and punished severely for refusing to surrender their opinions or activism. Nevertheless, there are many people with a great sense of responsibility standing in the frontline of this attack on all Palestinians, as well as an attack on the Arab and Muslim world. The organic and spontaneous resistance of Palestinian Jerusalemites has forced the soldiers to back off from Bab El-Amud and changed the pathway of the demonstration, postponed the High Court's decisions regarding the homes of Sheikh Jarrah, and brought about a large military drill to train soldiers in techniques to attack resistance groups.

There has been and there will be repercussions to what is taking place in Jerusalem. Gaza has caught the spark of freedom from Jerusalem. The distance to liberation nowadays is measured in reference to Jerusalem. So far, Gaza is closer to Jerusalem than Ramallah.

Gaza, the Betrayed

Originally published on *Middle East Monitor*, 28 January 2022

Gaza is less than 100 kilometres from Jerusalem. It is deliberately placed out of reach, separated by three visible borders. The Israeli border is the main obstacle, but there are two others, each affirming the authority of one of the two conflicting Palestinian factions: Ramallah's Palestinian Authority, and Gaza's own government. Less visibly, we are prevented from reaching Gaza by means of a diplomatic siege that has created institutional prohibitions. But even when official governmental permission to cross into Gaza is granted, we are often obligated to think of the institutional consequences.

Recently, after three attempts to enter Gaza on a medical mission, I managed to obtain all the right papers and to circumvent the institutional veto. I was contracted as a consultant by Medicins Du Monde (MDM) Spain to train and supervise psychologists working for the Ministry of Health and the Ministry of Education on the management of trauma-related conditions among children.

At the Erez checkpoint, the transition between the last Israeli neighbourhood in Ashkelon and the first Gazan neighbourhood of Beit Hanoun felt like a journey going back several decades in time. On the Israeli side, you see modern buildings, fancy cars and wide, modernised streets, while as you enter Gaza you are confronted with deteriorated infrastructure, broken roadways, carts drawn by animals, overcrowded living spaces, a multitude of children playing in the streets, dense lines of laundry hanging from the buildings, and fatigued faces regarding you with mysterious looks, perhaps wondering, "Why would anyone come to Gaza?"

To my surprise, there was no visible rubble of demolished homes remaining from the latest war on Gaza in May. I understood that any useful material is very quickly collected to be repurposed for future reconstruction. I noticed several amputee youth in the streets—young men and adolescents who lost a limb either during the war or because their knees were specifically targeted as they demonstrated in the Great March of Return. The graffiti displayed in the camps, in the city, and on the beach express support by the public of Gaza for Jerusalemites, for the people of Sheikh Jarrah, and for all Palestinian prisoners. *Gaza, the captive, expresses resistance in order to liberate us!*

War shines a spotlight on the misery of Gaza, but, very quickly, this misery falls back into oblivion. Today, as I sit in the warmth of home to write this article—benefitting from a day off work because of the snowstorm affecting the region—I learn of a baby in Khan Yunis who died from Gaza's lack of heating. Poverty, anaemia, food insecurity, lack of medical equipment, lack of fuel supply and lack of electricity are permanent in Gaza. I was deeply saddened when one of our trainees in Gaza, a senior colleague, mentioned in an informal gathering, "I visited Jerusalem last year." The colleagues in Gaza expressed curiosity and even envy—to explain, she added: "I am a cancer patient and I was granted permission to be treated at the Augusta Victoria Hospital." To have access to medical services outside Gaza one needs to be both very sick and very lucky at the same time.

Each of the clinical cases presented by the therapists was suffering from misery—in addition, in some instances, to psychopathology. Four out of 21 child cases were brought to supervision following the suicide of a family member. All of the others followed the traumatic death of a family member killed by the Israelis. In one case, the child was the only survivor of her family. In another case, the child's 17-year-old brother committed suicide after his mother pressured him to leave the home to obtain food; a sister reported to the school counselor that her mother was depressed and spent all of her time in bed. When a therapist reached out to the mother to offer support and an antidepressant, the mother responded: "I need food, not medication."

There is no safe place in Gaza. The face of trauma intrudes when a home is demolished, when a classmate is killed, when a cousin takes an illegal boat and disappears forever, when there is a threat of another war, and when Israel attacks the fishermen and the farmers to deter them from struggling to earn a living. The threats are many and real.

I left Gaza very early on a Sunday morning to catch up with my work in the West Bank. I encountered the endless line of Palestinian laborers waiting to cross the Erez checkpoint to work. I was told that they had been waiting since 4 am. In their lean bodies, dark wrinkled faces, cheap cigarettes and the plastic bags they carried with a change of underwear, I saw a tableau of modern slavery. Unlike them, I was unaware that the Israelis would not allow me to cross the checkpoint with my suitcase. I had to rush to empty its contents into plastic bags and throw away my suitcase before reaching the soldiers.

I went to Gaza to teach and supervise—but I learned a lot as a clinician, as a Palestinian compatriot and as a human being. If Gaza were one person, her deepest trauma would not be the enemy's aggression but the betrayal by her neighbours, her brothers and her sisters. We have yet to find a national remedy for this betrayal.

Gaza's New Mental Health Unit: A project of psychological control

Originally published on *Middle East Monitor*, 14 February 2020

In March, a field hospital being built by Israeli aid group Natan in conjunction with the American Evangelical Christian organisation Friend Ships will start operating in the northern Gaza Strip near the Erez crossing.

Authorities in occupied Ramallah claimed the project, spearheaded by pro-Israel donors, is a front for American and Israeli intelligence operations. PA Prime Minister Mohammed Shtayyeh accused the hospital of serving the Trump administration's "peace plan"; but unfortunately the protests were more to harm the public image of authorities in Gaza rather than to analyze and explain to Palestinians, including authorities in Gaza, the intended harm of such a project. In reaction, Hamas spokesman, Hazem Qassim, was defensive, telling Dunya Al-Watan: "They [the Palestinian Authority] wove them [their fears] together with imaginary information."

I have seen adverts calling for international volunteers including mental health professionals to work on the project, and discovered the following: Natan, an Israeli Tel Aviv based "non-profit humanitarian organisation", is part of this project, providing psychological care among other things, through non-Israeli passport holders contracted to provide health services in Gaza.

Friend Ships–Natan have also teamed up to provide medical care to Syrians on the Syrian-controlled side of the occupied Golan Heights.

In its call for volunteers, Natan said: "This new Health Center can directly influence Israeli security reducing the threat of violence from Gaza by improving the quality of life of the civilians there." The organisation uses mainstream Israeli language to describe Palestinians as a threat that needs to be controlled in every possible way, there is nothing about justice, occupation, or lifting the siege. In this instance, "improving the quality of life of civilians there" is a strategic method of control and hegemony.

The call especially mentions a member of Natan's Board, Major-General Matan Vilnai, former Deputy Chief of Staff of the Israeli army who is consulted to ensure the security of volunteers. The call does not mention however that this man has been charged with crimes against humanity over the 2009 bombing of Gaza. Nor does it mention his genocidal threats to Gazan "will bring upon themselves a bigger Shoah because we will use all our might to defend ourselves", using the Hebrew word normally reserved to refer to the Jewish Holocaust.

Staff and volunteers at the new medical center will enter the camp from Israel and the patients from the Palestinian side through checkpoints controlled by Israeli occupation forces chosen according to Vilnai's standards; so much for humanitarianism!

Israeli-supported American policies have undermined the health sector especially in Gaza. There is a major shortage in health care, medicines, and medical supplies that no one can deny. In appearance, the health care camp looks like an effort to mitigate these deliberate circumstances but in fact it is a way to impose more control and dependency on the most vulnerable among Palestinians.

Israel has negotiated with Palestinian patients hoping to leave the Gaza Strip for treatment, turning them into informants against their people in exchange for exit permits to access medical care. It has also prevented parents from accompanying their very sick children out of Gaza, leaving minors to die alone in Jerusalem hospitals.

Israel has imposed a siege, damaged infrastructure and caused a terrible humanitarian situation in Gaza, leaving it starving for aid and dependent on foreign humanitarian offerings. This has left those managing Gaza blind to the definite psychological and moral harm of this project, which allows Israel to wash its hands after all the blood it has spilt in the Strip and be both the perpetrator and the healer, exposing a very complex trauma dynamics.

An Israeli army-guarded health centre is the antithesis of a safe place required for psychological care. A volunteer therapist who accepts the premises of the project to improve the security of "Israel" and control Palestinian "violence" lacks the necessary awareness and the required empathy to be a therapist for Gazans; in fact, and at best, this is a project of improving public relations for Israel and granting a sizzling professional adventure for volunteers in a trauma zone.

Of course, there are other potential political and security risks of using this health complex; to tame the March or Return and wean genuine international solidarity that sends the Freedom Flotilla with a small amount of medical aid to Gaza. In a previous article I mentioned:

> a report from the UN Disengagement Observer Force (UNDOF) revealed that Israel has been collaborating with Salafi jihadi groups in the occupied Syrian Golan Heights; this collaboration was not restricted to offering medical aid to the injured members of Jabhat Al-Nusra. On the contrary, reports described the transfer of unspecified supplies from Israel to the Syrians, as well

as incidents when Israeli soldiers allowed free passage to Syrians who were not injured.

I'm afraid that this project will not only ship the material and equipment from the Syrian border to the Gaza border, but also the knowhow of using therapeutic rapport and medical intimacy to spy on the population, creating fractures and recruiting informants and collaborators.

On 11 November 2018, eight undercover Israeli agents disguised as members of a Palestinian family entered Gaza with the objective of planting listening devices on Hamas' private communications system. Investigations found the Israeli unit, which entered Gaza under the cover of international humanitarian organisation Humedica, a German-based body providing aid to Gaza, used spyware and drilling equipment.

Area Manager Joao Santos, who carried a Portuguese passport, fled Gaza a day after the operation failed. He is said to be a volunteer.

At a time when international politics is allowing Israel to have complete control over land and resources, humanitarianism is used to allow control of Palestinian minds. Humanitarianism can be a deceiving mask for sadistic intentions and maintaining the upper hand of Israelis over Palestinians. Promoting Palestinian self-sufficiency and ending the partition between Gaza and the West Bank immediately is the right response to this. Palestinian mental health professionals and services in the West Bank are eager to provide a response and meet the needs of those in Gaza as soon as our hands are freed.

Rescuing our Humanity from the Rubble of Gaza

The transcript of a talk given in Italy, November 2023

Every morning, we wake up to another horrific picture coming from Gaza: wild dogs eating the bodies of killed Gazans in Al Shifa hospital, a Palestinian's body dragged by a rope attached to an Israeli military vehicle near Zikim beach, forced nudity and torture imposed on Palestinian workers. Today, we saw the video of an Israeli tank ramming back and forth the corpse of a Palestinian civilian.

Respected audience: I'm a consultant psychiatrist, with long experience working with mental health professionals in Gaza. But I'm not here to talk to you about the unimaginable impact of genocide upon the mental health of Palestinians, or to romanticize the Palestinian Sumud. I'm here to warn you of the imminent collapse of our sense of common humanity. As a Palestinian without citizenship facing unprecedented levels of Israeli repression in Jerusalem and the West Bank, I call upon your universal principles as human beings to help us to expose the heart-wrenching reality unfolding in Gaza—a place that is being scarred by one of the darkest chapters in history. The relentless atrocities committed hour by hour in Gaza are a stain on humanity's conscience, leaving an indelible mark on our capacity to relate to one another as human beings.

Genocidal intent

From day one of this war, Israeli politicians have spoken vengefully of flattening Gaza and deporting its residents. The Israeli

Minister of Defense Yoav Gallant has described Gazans as "animals"; the President of Israel Isaac Herzog has declared that all Gazans are complicit in the acts of October 7th. These acts have been described as comparable to those of September 11th and Palestinian resistance fighters have been deemed comparable to ISIS—as if the events of October 7th marked the beginning of our history. The events of October 7th have been framed as if eight decades of occupation and repression of Palestinians had never taken place and as if there had not been two decades of imprisonment in Gaza, the largest contemporary concentration camp on earth. The Israeli Minister of Heritage Amichai Eliyahy has already remarked that dropping a nuclear weapon on Gaza is an "option". Baseless lies describing the beheading of Israeli babies and unfounded fiction of mass rape were invented to incite the world against Gaza and to legitimize the slaughter of its civilians.

Esteemed attendees, Israeli aerial bombardment has been relentless over the past 37 days of war. Through this, Gazan causalities in this single month have exceeded the total number of Ukranian causalities since the beginning of the war in Ukraine. Women and children account for 70% of Palestinian casualties. Kindly let that fact sink in—this is not simply a statistic, but a chilling testament to the intentional targeting of the most vulnerable. Medical staff, journalists, and civil defense forces are being targeted too. We behold people trying to rescue their family members from under the rubble with their bare hands and learn of doctors performing surgeries without anesthesia. Premature babies die because oxygen is cut off in hospitals. Many people in Gaza use their mobile phones to communicate their suffering to the world; we cannot claim that we didn't know. Live broadcast coverage of these massacres, spanning the entire past month, force the world to witness this horror, leaving no room for ambiguity about the identity of those responsible.

What is even more shocking to any sense of conscience is the unwavering support these massacres receive from the major Western regimes—the USA, UK, France, Germany and Italy. The blatant disregard for Palestinian life expressed by their political and military leadership, and in the mainstream Western media, contradicts the very values these nations claim to uphold. On the contrary, their disregard for the lives of Palestinians reveals the underlying racism and the colonial mentality of these Western regimes.

The infamous siege of Sarajevo serves as a stark comparison. At that time, the world witnessed the bombing of the Markale Market, resulting in 43 casualties, leading to NATO's decisive action against the Serbian forces. In contrast, Israel's bombing of the Baptist Hospital Al-Ahli, which resulted in the deaths of 500 civilians, met with Biden's hypocritical remark to Netanyahu, "it appears as though it was done by the other team". And Gaza is left to die of hunger, thirst, darkness, and lack of medical equipment.

Since 1948, the actions of the state of Israel have consistently breached international law. Shielded by unconditional support from the USA, Israel has considered itself immune to accountability. Yet these Western supported crimes against Palestinians are not just a violation of the rule of law, but a betrayal of our shared humanity. The deliberate onslaught by the Israeli government and military, fueled by its distorted sense of exceptionalism and revenge, is not only flattening Gaza; with every falling building, I see the moral collapse of the international community.

Dear comrades: as we know her, injured, aching, tearful and

feeling betrayed, Gaza will someday rise from the rubble and will look us in the eye. Perhaps she will ask us what role we played; perhaps she will simply forgive us as she has done many times before and will continue fighting the international world order alone. The urgency today lies in reviving our dying humanity, a humanity that has failed to preserve Gazan lives, foster compassion, and restore the values that define us as human beings. Let's rescue the remains of our humanity from the rubble of Gaza.

A Letter to Gaza Mental Health Professionals

Originally published on *USA Palestine Mental Health Network*, November 2023

Dear Mental Health Professionals in Gaza,

As we witness the impact of the war machine on the besieged territory of Gaza, we try to imagine the terrible psychological toll taken by its immense destruction and its traumatic losses of loved ones. It is only natural, and one suspects deliberate, that this devastation evokes in us a feeling of helplessness and hopelessness in applying our skills as mental health professionals.

What we confront is the futility of our tools and our work as professionals in the field of mental health. But we know that the savagery of this aggression has been designed to generate feelings of helplessness and guilt in our hearts, and to break the will of the Palestinian people. We also know that the role of mental health professionals can be a cornerstone in building hope and healing at every level of society. How can one escape bombings through relaxation exercises? How can we provide psychological first aid when there is no safe place, water, or food? How can we utilise digital means of psychosocial support when there is no internet connection?

This hope is also the ink in which the determination (Sumud) of everyone in solidarity around the world is being written. Your steadfastness, in particular, is the pillar of our resilience—as mental health professionals—whether in Palestine or anywhere on earth where the people aspire to freedom. You are the compass for those who are lost and a beacon in the darkness of despotism.

I am listening to the responses of the injured and the bereaved in Gaza, and I am amazed by the feelings of national unity and faith that they invoke to maintain their cohesion and resilience in adversity. Dear colleagues, build your psychological support on these concepts whenever they are evoked and reiterated. Use collective therapy and strategies of liberation psychology to enhance resilience and rebuild identity, thus contributing to the psychological recovery and well-being of the community. Despite the extent of destruction, we still have the capacity to maintain our mutual respect, interest, and empathy for one another.

My dear Gazans, colleagues contact me daily from Al-Quds [Jerusalem], the West Bank, the interior of the occupied country [Palestine '48], and from outside of Palestine, whether or not they are Arabs. They ask me how to help the people of Gaza—motivated as they are in solidarity with you during your terrible ordeal and hoping for your victory. The only thing preventing us from being directly by your side is the war machine that stands between us. We eagerly await the cessation of aggression to resume work with Gaza's institutions, its various organizations and humanitarian agencies, providing the necessary support and resources to strengthen the mental health of our people.

Finally, I would like to remind you, my dear colleagues, that you are not alone. All eyes see your faces, all ears listen to your words, and all hearts now beat to the rhythm of Gaza. You are martyrs and witnesses in this crucial stage of Palestinian and human history. Preserve the stories of people's lives, their dreams, and protect them as much as you can. Preserve the personal history of each of these individuals, their humanity, and their great courage in the face of desecration, as well as the history and rights of Palestinians in the face of tyranny. We will meet again soon, and we will work together to build better mental health services and help the people to recover and to rise. We are certain that our work as mental health professionals is a fundamental element in the project of national liberation in both of its aspects—liberating the human being and liberating the land.

With all my respect, and in the hope of a soonest liberation.

Dr Samah Jabr,
Consultant Psychiatrist
Director of Mental Health Unit, Palestinian Ministry of Health

Unmasking the False Generosity of the USA's Response to Gaza's Humanitarian Crisis

Originally published on *Middle East Monitor*, 18 March 2024

Amid dire warnings from the United Nations regarding the crisis of food insecurity in Gaza, the USA loudly proclaims to be delivering humanitarian aid to the region. But despite the impassioned remarks by Secretary of State Antony Blinken at the Davos summit, his recent visit to Israel yielded no substantial progress in increasing Palestinians' access to aid. Meanwhile, international leaders, echoing UN special rapporteurs, emphasize the size of the gravity of the situation—with reports indicating that widespread hunger is exacerbated by the Israeli actions targeting of the food system in Gaza.

We have already seen dozens of children and women dying of starvation, while those who are still living gaze with sunken eyes on an impotent world that does nothing to prevent the horrors they are enduring. Over six months, Israel has hampered deliveries of food, medical supplies and other aid items through the two land border crossings: Rafah with Egypt and Karem Abu Salem with the occupied land. Israeli inspections impede the flow of aid into Gaza Strip, with only a fraction of the required assistance reaching a small section of Palestinians.

Blocking aid is not a security need for the Israelis, but a strategic decision. As Knesset member Tali Gottlieb explained before that body on Oct 23, 2023:

Without hunger and thirst among the Gazan population, we will not be able to recruit collaborators, we will not be able to recruit intelligence, we will not be able to bribe people with food, drink, medicine in order to obtain intelligence; we know that finding the abductees is a supreme and super-important goal alongside the goals of fighting.

In response to rising criticism of Israel and its allies, US President Biden has announced his commitment to establish a floating harbor for aid delivery. The US conducted an airdrop of over 11,500 meals; some fell on the Israeli side, some in the sea, and others on the heads of starving people and killed them. The situation remains critical, with famine looming large over the Gaza Strip.

Despite these apparent acts of generosity, the underlying dynamics reveal a perpetuation of oppressive systems. This is a generosity that maintains the status quo benefiting the oppressor, while furthering the dependence of the oppressed. The actions taken by the USA, with all of its hypervisibility in international media, blur the capacity of the international onlookers to see the reality in Gaza. The appearance of generosity ignores and obscures the need to see clearly the ongoing challenges of addressing the root causes of the crisis and of ensuring sustainable relief efforts. Through the floating harbor, the US seems to be taking action, while simultaneously using its veto power to block ceasefire and giving a green light to the ongoing Israeli impediments to aid delivery. The harbor can be a project of control, rather than a project of humanitarian aid to Gazans.

The ongoing assault on Gaza has once again underscored the significant military assistance provided by the United States to Israel. The scale of military equipment dispatched to Israel during the conflict is staggering, with thousands of items, including bombs, artillery shells and drones being sent via numerous cargo planes and ships.

The financial aid provided by the US to Israel has always been substantial, totaling over $330 billion since 1948, with annual defense aid exceeding $3.8 billion. The recent passage of the USA's $95 billion foreign aid bill, with a significant portion allocated to Israel, further demonstrates its enduring commitment to support of the Israeli military. The recent self-immolation of a 25-year-old member of the US Air Force outside the Israeli Embassy in Washington, undertaken in protest against US complicity in genocide, is a tragic reminder of the extensive military aid received by Israel from its foremost ally.

Ever since October 7th, Israel has benefited from the USA's unwavering political, diplomatic and media support of the Israeli occupation. When meeting Israeli Prime Minister Benjamin Netanyahu in Tel Aviv, President Biden endorsed Israel's account of the attack on the Baptist hospital in Gaza by claiming, "It appears as though it was done by the other team."

The Israeli assault and Biden's reaction represented a litmus test of the international reaction to Israel's unprecedented attacks on Gaza's civilian population and its health system. US administration has repeatedly blocked Gaza ceasefire resolutions at the United Nations and bypassed Congress to increase weapons sales to Israel in a massive effort to enable Israel's path of destruction.

The USA's current humanitarian aid to Palestinians, offered in plain view of its longstanding support of Israel and its ongoing assistance to of the genocide in Gaza, is an embodiment of Paulo Freire's concept of "false generosity." To Freire, an act of false generosity addresses the symptoms of injustice without confronting its root causes—and, indeed, in the case of Israel, perhaps while nurturing the root causes. False generosity helps the giver, not the receiver. Biden's decision to provide humanitarian aid to Palestinians comes as he is running for re-election in November's presidential vote and it is perceived as an effort to appease the discontent within his Democratic Party's base regarding his steadfast backing of Israel's indiscriminate killing of civilians and destruction of hospitals, residential areas, and civilian structures.

True generosity, as articulated by Freire, involves addressing the systemic inequalities and power imbalances that sustain oppression. It requires a commitment to dismantling the structures that perpetuate poverty, hunger and suffering. Yet, the current approach of the USA, characterized by piecemeal aid efforts and simultaneous massive military support to Israel, falls far short of this transformative vision. This is pseudo-philanthropy providing only a semblance of humanitarian concern. In the case of the USA, true generosity would entail a genuine commitment to justice and liberation of Palestinian people; true generosity would entail promoting a ceasefire and meaningful peace-building efforts. Until then, the cycle of false generosity perpetuates the very injustices it claims to alleviate, serving the interests of the powerful while failing to address the needs of the oppressed.

Dignity Disguised: On the superficial meaning of humanitarian aid in Gaza

Originally published as 'The Indignities of Humanitarian Aid in Gaza' on *Mondoweiss*, 3 September 2024

Foreign organizations operating in Gaza, under the guise of "humanitarian" aid, distribute so-called "dignity kits", which include basic hygiene items like soap, sanitary pads, toothbrushes, and sometimes underwear. These organizations claim that their aim is to preserve the dignity of individuals, especially women and girls, during crises.

During a recent aid delivery from the British government to a field hospital in Gaza, Foreign Secretary David Cameron stated, "Many people in Gaza are suffering; no one should be without the basics of life like shelter and bedding, and everyone deserves the dignity provided by essential hygiene kits."

This statement, however, contrasts sharply with the UK's simultaneous support for Israel in its genocide against Palestinians in Gaza. This support includes assisting in military operations, implementing deals with Netanyahu's far-right government regarding joint trainings between British and Israeli military personnel, and providing intelligence services against Palestinians, as documented in multiple reports. British aircraft have conducted reconnaissance missions over Gaza, and Israeli military aircraft have visited Britain under undisclosed circumstances. Additionally, the UK facilitates US military support to Israel through its bases in Cyprus. This military alliance is coupled with Britain's commitment to defending Israel on the global stage against criticisms, particularly at the UN and in international legal forums. Despite these realities, media coverage often focuses on the distribution of dignity kits to Gazans, ignoring the broader context of Israeli actions against Palestinians.

This situation raises a critical question: How does war strip away dignity?

War begins by dehumanizing civilians through speech and actions that reduce them to mere objects in the eyes of aggressors, making the deprivation of their dignity seem acceptable. In Gaza, Israeli officials have likened Palestinians to animals and insects, an attempt to justify their oppression. War forces displacement, uprooting people from their homes and forcing them into overcrowded, degrading conditions, stripping them of control over their lives and deepening their dependence on external aid. Repeated displacements becoming the norm in Gaza have compounded this sense of lost dignity. War also breaks down family dynamics and the societal fabric that maintains cohesion, further deepening feelings of isolation and helplessness and moving the concept of dignity further away. In contrast to the aid receiving international attention, maintaining societal cohesiveness nurtures feelings of dignity.

War destroys essential infrastructure, such as hospitals, schools and water systems, robbing people of their right to meeting basic needs, and further eroding their quality of life. The targeting of healthcare facilities and the killing of medical workers in Gaza exemplify efforts not only to erase lives but also to obliterate the dignity that sustains them. Continuous exposure to violence and trauma—from home demolitions and shelling to constant surveillance—breeds pervasive fear and insecurity, undermining psychological stability and stripping individuals of the basic sense of security integral to human dignity.

The problem with "dignity kits" in Gaza is multifaceted:

- Double Standards and Complicity: The distribution of dignity kits by governments and organizations that contribute to or are complicit in the ongoing siege and violence against Gaza is a glaring contradiction. These entities, while claiming to uphold dignity, are instrumental in creating the conditions that strip Gaza's people of their humanity and dignity. The distribution of these kits serves as a superficial gesture that obscures their role in perpetuating the root causes of suffering, almost as a means to console the Western conscience by providing some soap to those enduring constant violence.

- Reducing Dignity to Material Items: The notion that dignity can be preserved or restored through basic hygiene items is deeply troubling. Offering soap to those whose families have been killed and homes destroyed trivializes the concept of dignity, reducing it to mere bodily cleanliness while ignoring the profound psychological and emotional wounds inflicted by injustice. True dignity is an integral feeling that surpasses material items; it encompasses self-respect, human worth, and the ability to live freely and independently. For the people of Gaza, dignity is inextricably linked to liberation from violence and occupation, the right to self-determination, and access to essential services without dependency on external aid. Providing material goods should not replace support for the Palestinian resistance against genocide. This approach does not address the deeper needs of Gazans or Palestinians and can be seen as an attempt to assuage Western guilt while ignoring ongoing violations of Palestinian rights.

- Gender Discrimination: The focus on women in the distribution of dignity kits often reflects a Western-imposed sensitivity that overlooks the suffering of men, especially those involved in resistance. Women are often portrayed as helpless victims in need of special protection, while men, particularly Arab Muslim resistance fighters, are either ignored or depicted as less deserving of empathy. This reinforces traditional stereotypes and excludes men from receiving necessary care, further entrenching gender divisions—as if men are to blame for bringing war upon themselves and other women, which exempts them from Western empathy and dignity kits. True justice requires a comprehensive approach that supports both women and men, recognizing their individual and collective needs.

In conclusion, the extent of Gazan suffering, from the obliteration of security and privacy in crowded conditions of constant displacement, makes even basic needs like using the bathroom or eating difficult. While dignity kits may provide immediate relief, they are no substitute for true dignity, which can only be restored through liberation from oppression. The term "dignity kits" in Gaza is misleading and superficial, diminishing the profound struggle that Palestinians are engaged in for their freedom. True dignity is not granted through material items but achieved through the end of violence and the recognition of Palestinians' rights to self-determination and justice. In Gaza, dignity is a collective value representing the right of the Palestinian people to live in freedom and security. Any attempt to restore dignity through material goods is an arrogant oversimplification of a much deeper struggle.

Family in Palestine

How Israel Exploits Gender Roles to Discredit Palestinian Female Activists

Originally published on *Middle East Eye*, 29 May 2020

In *A Dying Colonialism,* Frantz Fanon describes the French colonial mindset in Algeria: "If we want to destroy the structure of Algerian society, its capacity for resistance, we must first of all conquer the women; we must go and find them behind the veil where they hide themselves and in the houses where the men keep them out of sight."

In Palestine, Israel's oppression of men and women differs in impact. Men are exposed to occupation-related violence due to their greater presence in the public sphere, while women are targeted in other ways. Oppression and colonialism exacerbate pre-existing gender inequalities, as political violence encourages a "protective" attitude that hinders women from participation in community life.

The occupation undermines the masculinity of Palestinian men by humiliating and belittling them. A man whose dignity is assaulted at a checkpoint can easily displace the sense of defeat onto one weaker than himself, often a woman at home.

Inciting scorn

The pervasive impoverishment of families under occupation, and the sense of a bleak future, encourages early marriage for girls and dropping out of school for boys.

Women are further insulted as Israeli politicians describe their wombs as demographic time bombs, as the Palestinian birth rate soars. This prejudice can impede the access of pregnant women to hospitals, causing them to give birth at checkpoints, with tragic death rates for both the infants and their mothers, as reported by the *Lancet*.

Gendered tactics are also commonly used to discredit Palestinian female activists, stripping them of their femininity and social standing, and inciting men to scorn them.

A 2018 Facebook post by a spokesperson for the Israeli occupation army, for example, included the following message alongside a picture of a female demonstrator from Gaza: "The good woman is the honourable woman, who takes care of her home and her children, and serves as a good example to them. However, the deprived woman who lacks honour does not take care of these things, acts wildly against her feminine nature, and cares not for how she is seen in society."

Commenting on the honour and "natural" role of women reinforces inequitable gender stereotypes and deters women from political action. Societies and families are thus reminded to limit women to "traditional" roles to protect them from violence and abuse.

Political prisoners

The gender discrepancy is perhaps greatest, however, in the experience of political prisoners. I work with female former prisoners to assist with psychological care and legal documentation, and it has taught me a lot about how the Israeli military system uses gendered tactics and insinuations of cultural taboos to apply pressure on female prisoners and broader Palestinian society.

During decades of Israeli occupation, thousands of Palestinian women have been arrested; like men, they are jailed for their activism or detained to inflict pressure on activist relatives. Sometimes, the cries of a woman under "interrogation" are used to force her brother, husband, or son to confess.

Last summer, Mais Abu Ghosh, a university student, was tortured for a month; when her parents were brought to the interrogation centre, they could not recognise her. Strip searches and exchanging sanitary pads and toilet paper for information are common practices, to which many women prisoners have been exposed.

Imprisoned women especially suffer from the destruction of their social ties, often being held outside the 1967-occupied territory, in contravention of Article 76 of the Fourth Geneva Convention. Their relatives are often denied the necessary permits to visit them.

Female prisoners are also denied psychological help when they need it most. In January 2018, Israa Jaabis, a Palestinian mother from Jerusalem charged with attempted murder after her car exploded near an Israeli checkpoint in 2015, wrote a painful letter complaining that prison authorities deprived her from seeing her son, and expressing her great need of psychological help.

"I feel scared when I look at my face in the mirror, so imagine what others must feel when they look at me," she wrote, noting that her medical and psychological needs were neglected, despite UN rules stating that prison authorities "shall endeavour to ensure that [female prisoners have] immediate access to specialised psychological support or counselling".

Female prisoners also suffer from what takes place outside prison. Whenever a man is jailed, there is very often an over-extended woman compensating for his absence; but when a woman is put behind bars, her motherhood is questioned and her husband pressed to find a new wife to provide "a mother for his children".

Although not uttered openly, the view persists that a female prisoner is reprehensible for leaving her children behind. A loud silence surrounds the possibility that she has been sexually assaulted in custody.

While Palestinian men are generally glorified after being released from prison, women in the same situation face further struggles to find a job, connect with a partner, and assume an active role in an increasingly "protective" society.

Structural violence

Oppression in Palestine has many fronts, through which structural violence and political repression hinder people's liberties and freedom. Women—especially activists and former prisoners—face a multitude of intersecting struggles in their journey towards liberation.

Feminist movements have shied away from advocating for the rights of Palestinian female prisoners, but it is these sources of power that can expose the gendered dimensions of the occupation in Palestine and ensure these inequalities and systems of oppression are not overlooked.

Palestinians should challenge such dynamics, which weaken our capacity to resist the occupation and subjugate us further. Gender divides power. Women's lack of influence contributes to colonialism and other ethnic-class power relations.

More flexibility in gender roles would increase the resilience of Palestinians in the face of trauma, freeing women from the prison within so that they can become active agents of change and resistance.

There Is No Father: Palestinian adolescents stand tall for liberation

Originally published on *Middle East Eye*, 27 October 2015

The self-inspired and improvized participation of adolescents who have no political affiliation is a remarkable phenomenon in this current uprising. These are the minors who were born after the Oslo Accords and watched at a distance the three wars upon Gaza, who witnessed the settlers' growing viciousness against our villagers in the West Bank, and who now see clearly the Israeli expansion currently taking over all that is Palestinian in Jerusalem.

These boys are neither desperate nor suicidal, nor are they delinquent and immoral offenders. On the contrary, the biographies of many of them display an ambitious striving for excellence and achievement. They perceive themselves as capable, altruistic and protective of the Palestinian people—and are willing to endure extreme sacrifices to realize these goals.

Ahmad Manasra, 13, was injured by Israelis and left to bleed on the light train railway, accompanied by obscene shouts by Israeli by-passers to "give him a bullet in the head" in retaliation for accusations that he stabbed an Israeli youth. This youngster was a student at Al Nayzak, enrolled in an extra-curricular programme for students talented in science, technology, engineering and maths.

Mustafa Al Khatib, 17, was a popular and distinguished student at the Al Ibrahimeyeh School. But the childhoods of these children are completely unacknowledged by the Israelis, whose media report the day following the event was entitled: "13 Year Old Terrorist Stabbed a 13 Year Old Boy."

I do not seek to encourage violence, but I am driven to understand and to explain its origins and to call for an adult response to it. Adolescence is a developmental phase normally characterized by impulsivity, emotional lability and a search for identity. Our adolescents don't pass through this phase peacefully however. "We will take you to room Number Four. Do you know what that is? You enter it on two legs but come out on all fours."

This testimony has been reported frequently following the Israeli interrogation of minors in the Russian compound in Jerusalem over recent years—well before the current clashes. This is the Israelis' strategic goal for Palestinians living under occupation, to objectify and exploit them as animals on all fours, gazing at the ground, who do not dare to stand up for their rights. "The only good Arab is a dead Arab" is a slogan often repeated by Israelis in expressing the majority's sentiments towards Palestinians.

Today we are seeing these "dead Arabs" and these "Palestinians on all fours" stand up against the enduring violation and intimidation of their people and attack their oppressor with primitive weapons. In so doing, they reassert in extreme form that they have will and agency, that they are capable of making choices, and that they are willing to risk a likely death by standing up to the enemy. What they are not willing to do is to live "on all fours".

Over the years, the occupation has undermined the structure of Palestinian families and disorganized its community. Palestinian fathers are weakened, unable to provide for their families or to protect them from injury. Eighty per cent of Jerusalem residents live below the poverty line, in inadequate and unhealthy housing, with a "temporary residency" status that can be revoked for the slightest perceived defiance of the occupation. Drug addiction is a growing problem. There are dramatically visible discrepancies in life-style and opportunities between East and West Jerusalem. The more they breathe freely in West Jerusalem, they more we choke in East Jerusalem.

Many Palestinian fathers were killed or made psychologically absent by imprisonment or the trauma of torture; one third of all Palestinian men have been in Israeli detention at one time or another since 1967. Many of these fathers, released after long years in prison, have become shadows of their previous selves. These fathers observe that their eldest sons, although in fact mere adolescents, have become the "father" in their place.

Our children often experience the arrest of a child in their home. They behold their fathers standing helpless as the masked Israeli soldiers burst in with their military dogs, shouting at the family in Hebrew as a young sibling is snatched from his bed. In some cases, fathers were forced to hand over their children to the soldiers while swallowing their tears. They witnessed their mothers beaten, humiliated and undressed when they too tried to defend their children, and saw their paralyzed father unable to protect her. Falah Abu Maria, from Beit Ummar, was killed when he tried to defend his son from soldiers in July.

In addition, these children have only experienced an abusive and unsuccessful Palestinian leadership. After the Palestinian parliamentary elections in 2006, the Palestinian president rationalized the rejection of its outcome by saying "if we have to choose between bread and democracy, we choose bread". Just before last summer's war in Gaza, this president informed the Palestinians that "security coordination with Israel is sacred". And recently, at the opening session of the Palestinian National Council, he made the outrageous assertion: "We have nothing to do with Jerusalem,

the Prophet has left Mecca." The Palestinian leadership has permitted the suffocating siege in Gaza and worked in coordination
with Egypt and Israel to flood the tunnels around it. Recently the
Palestinian leadership has arrested every Palestinian who possesses
the potential to stand up to settlers in the West Bank and has
brutally repressed peaceful demonstrations opposing the Israeli
attacks on the Al Aqsa mosque.

Israel has deliberately attacked and discredited anyone who
might play the role of a positive father figure in the eyes of
Palestinians. Many Palestinian leaders have been assassinated by
Israeli forces; the Palestinian minister Zeyad Abu Ein died in violent confrontation with soldiers; a Palestinian judge was killed
at a checkpoint under disputed circumstances, and the entire
Israeli Arab leadership is intimidated and threatened with expulsion. Israel has detained dozens of members of the Palestinian
Legislative Council and gone so far as to propose body searches of
Arab Knesset members before they enter the Knesset in order to
further debase the image of the Palestinian leadership.

Palestinian adolescents know very well that they have an
extremely limited personal future under occupation, with its
forced imposition of desperate economic, political and social
conditions. But it is the promise of "the future" that helps developing children and youths postpone their natural impulsiveness
and submit to the guidance of their parents. Foreseeing nothing
but their wasted potential ahead of them, Palestinian adolescents
are robbed of the incentives to rein in the age-appropriate recklessness and impulsiveness of adolescence. Perceiving themselves
as having nothing to lose and no one upon whom to model themselves, they are vulnerable to a concrete identification with the

massive trauma, violence, bereavement and death all around them.

The occupation with its shattered dreams both magnifies and masks all other forms of adolescent aspiration and adolescent suffering. The violent involvement in resistance to the occupation among these youths is a symptom of the disorganisation of the society in which they are struggling to survive. And Palestinian adults, often having succumbed to humiliation, fear and learned helplessness, have failed to meet these fearless but fatherless children half way; we have left behind a void by failing to rise to the challenge of our responsibilities.

The confrontation between the occupied and the occupier is the natural outcome of the Palestinian reality—far more so than the typical official false submission to the Israelis punctuated by occasional outbursts against them. Our leadership has failed to set an agenda and a national strategy for liberation; it has avoided and feared the process of raising Palestinian awareness and prohibited the development of both authentic discourse and the provision of genuine tools for liberation.

Our leadership has failed to promote education as a vehicle for our dignity and neglected the task of healing the trauma of humiliation. Instead, our leaders have encouraged factional chauvinism, polarisation, corruption and nepotism, and distributed favours on the basis of compliance and political affiliation.

The acts of our youth express a valid and legitimate yearning for freedom and dignity, but this yearning needs our support and nurturing. We must protect our youth from a recklessness that can abort their lives and their goal—as will happen in the absence of the positive boundaries, limit-setting, and social values that fatherly leadership provides.

The spontaneous reaction of our children to the occupation should be a warning of the need for fundamental political reform in Palestine, alerting us to the need to survive as individuals and to thrive as a nation. Their actions should be a wake-up call for us as adults, a catalyst to organize a truly meaningful project to end the occupation.

Arrested Adolescence: On the interrupted development of Palestinian minors in prison

This article was published on *Samidoun: Palestinian Prisoner Solidarity Network*, 17 January 2016

The Israeli parliament has recently approved a law that allows the sentencing of up to 20 years in prison for Palestinians who throw stones, for individuals who are usually minors. This development was followed by a law that would allow for the imprisonment of Palestinian children as young as 12, if they are found guilty of "nationalistically-motivated" violent offences.

As a clinician, I am often confronted with adolescents whose social and psychological growth has been suspended by experiences of political detention. I observe that many such youths have become anxious and depressed following this experience, whereas others manifest stoicism and fail to express any emotion.

"Majed" (all names have been changed) is a boy of 14; he has been arrested 14 times and often beaten brutally in detention. On one occasion, the Israeli forces broke his teeth and inflicted a number of head injuries. Majed was brought to my clinic by an older sister who had just finished medical school. She explained that he did not listen to anyone at home, no longer respected his teachers, and frequently missed school. Instead, he befriended men of 30 or 40 and accompanied them to spend time in coffee shops. I found in Majed an adolescent experiencing a hypertrophic growth of his status as a hero, at the expense of compromising other areas of personality development. This profile of adolescent ex-detainees is typical. Less commonly, we see reactions such as that of Mufeed, in whom the experience of detention brought a deeper destruction, at least with regard to his image of his father. Mufeed claimed that "the prison guard was better than my father; he gave me cigarettes to smoke".

Majed and Mufeed are just two among the 700 Palestinian youths arrested each year. The average age of arrest is 15 and the average duration of their detention in prison is 147 days. Ninety per cent of these minors have been documented as having been exposed to traumatic experiences and 65 of them have developed diagnosable psychiatric disorders. For these minors and adolescents, the experience of arrest is superimposed upon a childhood already rendered difficult due to the Israeli occupation, in which social services and educational support systems are poor, nutrition and health care are inadequate, and political violence is rampant.

Adolescence everywhere is characterized by an accelerated movement towards social independence and identity formation, as well as by emotional lability and impulsive behaviour. However, the context of the occupation makes the risks greater and the consequences heavier for Palestinian adolescents. Some youngsters find the dangers inherent to resistance to be more exciting than a passive surrender to oppression. Such young people empathize and identify with the suffering of the community as a group and seek to establish a special status for themselves by acting on its behalf. While adolescents elsewhere may romanticize and model themselves on media stars, some Palestinian adolescents romanticize freedom fighters, like the figure of Muhannad Elhalaby, who countered his sense of helplessness by grabbing the gun of an Israeli settler and killing two settlers in the midst of attacks on the mosque.

The reality of detention is a story of horror, helplessness and humiliation for minors. It is usual for dozens of armed soldiers and their dogs to invade the family home in the middle of the night, interrupting the sleep of the whole neighbourhood and demonstrating through their excessive aggression that resistance is meaningless. The child's father is intimidated through threats to hand over his boy to the soldiers, and often does so despite the tearful pleas of the mother and siblings. Snatched in this way from his warm bed, the boy is exposed to unnecessary disorientation and physical violence as he is transferred to an unknown destination, often for an unknown reason as well. Typically he is handcuffed painfully and blindfolded, unable meanwhile to communicate with or to understand people who are shouting at him in Hebrew. He is slapped, kicked, punched and shoved as he is tied up and rendered completely powerless. Then, without a lawyer or a parent present, he is interrogated for a period of time extending from hours to weeks, with deprivation of relief for physiological needs such as the availability of food, drink, toilet facilities and sleep. He is exposed to excessive heat or cold, forced into the horror of witnessing others being tortured, and stripped naked before being subject to the same procedures himself.

Interrogators inflict guilt by threats made to his family members: "We will bring your mother and sisters here" and "We will demolish your home." Leaving the horror to the child's imagination, the interrogator might play with a rubber glove while telling the minor, "If you don't tell us the names of your friends who throw stones, something really bad will happen to you." Detained youngsters are often told that their friends or neighbours have already informed on them and many break down in response to this lie; they end up signing their names to Hebrew documents that they are not able to read. Many such children and adolescents recall these moments especially with unbearable feelings of shame. These youngsters are then relegated to isolation and uncertainty within the hostile prison environment, where the passage of time and life processes are frozen. Here their human attachments are destroyed, as few families succeed in gaining permission to visit their children.

In March 2013, during a period of relative political calm, the United Nations Children's Fund (UNICEF) described the ill-treatment of Palestinian minors held in Israeli military detention centres as "widespread, systematic and institutionalised". UNICEF examined the Israeli military court system and found evidence of "cruel, inhuman and degrading treatment or punishment". There are reports of circumstances in which dogs were utilized to attack children; where children and adolescents were sexually violated; and where youngsters were forced to witness or to perform acts that degraded their religious symbols.

The process of arresting minors targets the future of the Palestinian nation. It is an attack on the body, the personality, the belief system, the hopes and the dreams of young Palestinians, rendering their families dysfunctional and breaking the bonds of their connection with their community.

Many of these minors emerge from prison unable to learn in school or to pursue a profession. In their eyes, their parents and teachers are damaged as authority figures. Their trust in their friends and neighbours is destroyed. Their own community may not trust them either, because other children would have been told that they had implicated them to their interrogators. They live with the ongoing and realistic fear of further detention. And the family often experiences the arrest of the minor as extremely traumatic; they feel guilty for failing to protect him and thereby may indeed grow incapable of guiding the minor in a safe journey from childhood to adulthood. Unable to develop, left without education or family guidance, many adolescents thus fail to develop a mature and multifaceted adult identity. The ex-detainee clings to his identity as a prisoner. Such youngsters are stuck in perpetual limbo, unable to return to the innocence of childhood or to move forward as functional adults.

A feeling of ineffectiveness often seeps into clinicians who treat these youngsters. The psychological consequences of minors' arrest do not lend themselves to diagnostic labelling, pathologizing and medicalizing. These youngsters require us to act as witnesses, to join them in solidarity and to accompany them and their families in the exploration of the meaning of experience. It is our goal to help them reprocess this meaning, and to integrate it into their current life and in their plans for the future.

Hippocrates told doctors 25 centuries ago that we are not often able to cure; that we are sometimes able to treat; but that we are always able to offer comfort. We, clinicians, cannot liberate these children from Israeli prisons, but we may succeed in liberating them from the prison within as they come back to our community.

In Palestine, a Growing Sense of Alienation Pervades Society

Originally published on *Middle East Eye*, 2 April 2019

The international consensus is moving towards new laws criminalizing non-violent opposition to Zionism as 'anti-semitism'.

The current world offers countless examples of alienation, but this phenomenon is perhaps especially commonplace in Palestine.

I recently observed a prestigious professional meeting, in which a well-regarded woman dared to defend her opinion with technical data and logic against the meeting's "boss" and the massive wall of silence his presence evoked (the boss being not a technical person himself, but someone with political power).

Trying to discredit her remarks, the boss said: "This is Abu Antar talking!" He was referring to a male character within the Arab media. Abu Antar is a popular, muscular and defiant gangster. The comment by the boss can be understood as meaning it is not "womanly" to be defiant and protest. The woman responded: "Only someone unsure of his own masculinity would need to utter such a comment."

The need to belong

Those present—including a number of women appointed merely to appease the project donor's gender policy, and who fill the role of Amen-sayers to whatever the boss happens to utter—promptly sighed in collective disapproval at the woman's shrewd reply.

In my discipline of psychiatry, the need to belong is placed high on Maslow's hierarchy. Group identity is viewed by psychologist

Erik Erikson as a crucial psychosocial developmental stage, without which people feel alienated.

Alienation has been assumed to be the root cause of mass shootings in the US, a motivator for people to follow the Islamic State, and a driver of risky migration practices.

The phenomenon of alienation represents an intersection of the personal and the collective, the psychological and the sociological. It includes feelings of powerlessness, meaninglessness and self-estrangement.

Alienation can be generated by design: in Palestine, pervasive political helplessness and economic misery alienates many from one another. "I rarely see my children," noted a labourer at an Israeli border checkpoint. "By the time I return home, they are already in bed getting their rest for school the next morning."

Palestinians are alienated from their land and from international consciousness. Forgotten is United Nations General Assembly Resolution 3379, which identified Zionism as a form of racism. Instead, the international consensus is moving towards new laws criminalizing non-violent opposition to Zionism as "anti-semitism".

Reframing enemies and friends

Recent events have accelerated and generalized Palestinians' sense of alienation from the traditionally supportive Arab–Muslim community.

The latest Warsaw conference on Middle East "peace", attended by Arab leaders and Israel's Benjamin Netanyahu, reframed enemies and friends, resulting in the Gulf states crowning Israel as a leader in their fight against Iran and ignoring the occupation of Palestine.

US policy in the Middle East is based on efforts to normalize relations between Israel and the Arab world, fuelled by the rise of Arab leaders who are shamelessly willing to sacrifice the Palestinian cause, while the Arab people are exhausted in revolutionary struggles against their leaders.

All of these developments are changing norms and further isolating Palestinians.

Rapid growth in the relationship between Israel and Arab governments, especially in the Gulf, has been manifested through official visits by senior Israeli officials to Arab countries, such as Prime Minister Netanyahu's visit to Oman last November. There has also been an expansion of informal meetings and a flurry of economic activity between Arab and Israeli companies.

All of this is accompanied by the artificial support of cyber trolls on social media, aiming to create a false public opinion in support of normalization in Arab society—an accelerated process of spiritual and symbolic degradation. In reality, this transformation is limited to the leaders and political elites in the Arab world. Ordinary citizens and public opinion steadfastly oppose normalization with Israel.

Grassroots movements on the Arab street, and their aspirations to be freed from regime control, reveal the degree to which public opinion has been falsified.

Backing oppressive regimes
Israel is the enemy of the Arab people wherever they may be, backing their oppressive regimes, monitoring their activists, and aiding the process of human rights violations. For example, an Israeli company specializing in cyber-espionage reportedly

negotiated a multimillion-dollar deal with Saudi Arabia for technology that could be used to hack dissidents' mobile phones.

The Palestinian leadership, which allows for security coordination with Israel, has paved the way for the normalization between Israel and Arab regimes. This disappointment is exacerbated by the widespread polarization, corruption and nepotism practiced by Palestinian leaders and institutions.

Yet, there are still examples of resistance to this alienation. A photo recently emerged of Hebron's police chief helping to change a flat tyre on an Israeli military jeep, sparking widespread rage among Palestinians and eventually leading to the chief's suspension.

These are difficult times, indeed. The alienated are many and silent. But we shall hold on; we will not disappear. We shall speak about the ills of alienation. Sometimes this will cause further pain, and sometimes it will expose the collaborators—but this is what it takes to walk the road of freedom, for our minds and our homeland.

Innocence Under Fire: The deepening crisis for Gaza's children and their cry for help

Originally published on *Middle East Monitor*, 18 March 2024

Amid the relentless military onslaught by Israel on the Gaza Strip, the plight of children in this besieged region worsens by the day. The need for psychological and social support for these young souls was evident even before the current escalation, but now it has reached a critical juncture.

In the words of António Guterres, the Secretary-General of the United Nations, Gaza has tragically transformed into a grave-yard for children. Shockingly, approximately 17,000 children in Gaza are left without the care of their families or are separated from them, intensifying their psychological and social anguish. Doctors on the ground have coined a grim acronym, "WCNSF", for "wounded child, no surviving family", highlighting the heart-wrenching reality faced by countless children. Each day, dozens of children endure amputations, leaving them with permanent disa-bilities, while the specter of famine looms large, exacerbating an already dire situation of malnutrition and anemia.

The violence ravaging Gaza inflicts deep psychological wounds on its children, who urgently require support to navigate the daily horrors they endure. As their numbers in need of assistance grow, the challenge becomes increasingly daunting and complex.

UNICEF underscores the critical necessity of providing psycho-logical, social and emotional support to all children facing severe violence in Gaza. Yet, the consequences of war extend far beyond the immediate, casting a long shadow over their future. The trauma they endure threatens to erode their trust in the world, shatter their sense of purpose, and hinder their ability to connect with others and themselves, fostering a pervasive sense of insecurity that may haunt them for life.

Children, in their tender years of development, are uniquely vulnerable to the psychological toll of war. Their cognitive and emotional faculties are still maturing, rendering them ill-equipped to process the horrors they witness. They lean heavily on their caregivers for solace and security, but when these pillars falter under the weight of war's trauma, children are left adrift in a sea of fear and abandonment.

Moreover, their limited understanding of the conflict compounds their distress, leaving them grappling with confusion and helplessness. Disruptions to their routines, coupled with exposure to the harrowing sights, sounds and smells of war, further exacerbate their anguish, triggering intense emotional reactions and deepening their psychological scars. We noticed a girl freezing at the sound of thunder, and a boy exhibiting severe anxiety as he talks about seeing a tank.

The humanitarian crisis facing Gaza's children demands urgent intervention from the international community and humanitarian organizations. Their innocence, combined with their dependence on caregivers and the relentless onslaught of war, leaves them uniquely vulnerable. It is imperative that we prioritize their well-being, offering them the support and resources they need not only to survive but to recover and thrive amid the rubble of Gaza. Their cries for help must not go unheard, for they represent the hope and future of a generation caught in the fire of genocide.

Understanding Palestine's Colonial, Intergenerational Trauma from a Mental Health Perspective

Interview originally published on *The Hindu*, Saumya Kalia, 16 November 2023

In Palestine, trauma does not sit alone with the individual, and it does not lie idle in the past. Millions of people in a densely populated sliver of land are facing a persistent loss of home, land and safety. One out of 200 people has died in Gaza since October 7. Every hour, on average, 42 Israeli bombs fall, 12 buildings are levelled, 15 people are killed (six of them children), and 35 are injured as per United Nations OCHA data. Water, food, fuel and electricity have run out inside hospitals and across the region, triggering an unprecedented humanitarian crisis.

The late Eyad El-Sarraj, founder of the Gaza Community Mental Health Programme, said in 2005 that the psychological effects of Israel's occupation of Gaza, and of violence in Palestine, have created a "learned helplessness". The aim is "making the whole population captive to fear and paralysis".

Q: Studies show post-traumatic (PTSD) is among the most commonly recognized psychological disorders among Palestinians. You have previously questioned the methodology of these studies—they measured "social psychological pain and social suffering". What was the nature of your concerns with this?

A: The concern might involve both the methodology and the way trauma is articulated. Studies measuring "social psychological pain and social suffering" might capture the broader societal impact of trauma, but could potentially overlook individual experiences and the complexity of trauma responses. On the other hand, an individualistic approach to trauma might pathologize the individual and fail to provide solutions to the pathologizing context. Trauma in the Palestinian context is a complex and deeply layered topic. In my clinical practice, I more often see people affected by a prolonged, enduring collective trauma that changed their world outlook and belief systems as compared to people who suffer from the usual reexperiencing, hypervigilance and avoidance symptoms of PTSD.

Q: You wrote Palestinians often use this phrase to describe their feelings: '*Badany Masmoum, Maqhour, Mazloum, Maksour Khatry.*' (I feel that my body is intoxicated, oppressed, exposed to injustice; my desire is broken.) What do you see, and hear, from people who have lived under a regime of discrimination and violence for decades?

A: Palestinians have been exposed to chronic stressors, including grief, displacement, economic hardship, and the ongoing threat of detention. The phrase you mentioned encapsulates a profound sense of physical and emotional distress, and cognitive changes, reflecting an ongoing suffering and psychological impact. The psychological impact of shattered hopes, dreams, and aspirations; of feeling abandoned and betrayed. It represents the breakdown of personal aspirations and the collective yearning for a peaceful and dignified life amid the persistent conflict. Over time, Palestinian expressions of trauma have likely evolved due to prolonged exposure to conflict and oppression. This exposure over generations has not only led to adaptive responses, but also significant psychological distress, which affects their cognitive processes, emotional regulation, and interpersonal relationships. Living under such conditions for an extended period can lead to a range of psychological impacts: heightened anxiety, depression, feeling helpless. Moreover, prolonged exposure to trauma can alter brain development in children and drain functions in adults, impacting memory, attention, and decision-making processes. It can change the personality, identity, the view of self and others.

Q: Can you explain the intergenerational mental health impact of Israel's policies? The segregation or the chronic underinvestment in infrastructures? How do families process this routine discrimination?

A: Oppressive policies, displacement, and denial of homes have long-lasting effects on families and generations. The absence of a stable home environment and chronic stressors impact mental health across generations. Trauma will not only affect the attachment between a parent and a child, but also a traumatized parent can pass it on (epigenetics) to the offspring. There are endless examples of this [intergenerational trauma]. Look at Palestinians' reaction to all these calls to displace people in Gaza. Because we have a history of displacement and the Nakba, the reaction to images of people being dispossessed from their homes in Gaza is of a continous fear.

Q: Can you explain your criticism of post-traumatic stress disorder (PTSD) or the Beck inventory as Western, colonial concepts? What has shaped our understanding of "trauma" and psychological distress today?

A: You're absolutely correct that Western mental health tools and diagnostic criteria, such as those used for PTSD, often fall short of understanding and addressing the experiences of non-Western or marginalized communities. They rely on cultural frameworks, which might not adequately consider the complexities of cultural nuances, historical contexts, and the collective nature of trauma prevalent in societies like Palestine.

In many non-Western cultures, the expression of distress or trauma might differ significantly from what is outlined in standardized diagnostic manuals. For instance, in Palestinian culture, the experience of trauma might be expressed through somatic symptoms, communal storytelling, or religious/spiritual explanations rather than fitting neatly into the symptom categories defined by Western psychiatric criteria. Mental health issues in communities like Palestine are often deeply intertwined with the region's historical and ongoing political turmoil, such as displacement, occupation and oppression, affecting entire communities rather than just individuals—and with this comes a feeling of normalcy. Western tools may overlook the socio-political influences (which are determinants of mental health), failing to capture the full scope of trauma experienced collectively.

Also, the therapeutic interventions might be inappropriate: suggesting self care for a people facing genocide is not a good idea! In collectivist societies like Palestine, trauma is often shared collectively among families, neighbourhoods, or entire communities. This collective nature of trauma might not align with the individualized focus of Western diagnostic criteria. Traumatic experiences, such as the loss of land, displacement, or witnessing violence against family members, can have far-reaching effects that extend beyond individual psychological symptoms.

Q: Israel is attacking schools and healthcare facilities like Al Shifa Hospital—where patients, civilians, journalists and aid workers are taking refuge—indiscriminately. How does the brain, the body and the person respond to a continued denial of safety?

A: A prolonged lack of safety can lead to chronic stress, affecting both the brain and the body. Constant exposure to danger triggers heightened stress responses, impacting mental health and well-being. Usually, stress responses include physiological responses—like shortness of breath, headaches, stomachaches, and numbness in the limbs. It can be any physiological response—somatosensory and aches and pains.

But it is impossible to provide useful mental health interventions when there is no safe place.*

Q: How would you differentiate between "individual" trauma and "collective" trauma? For instance, how would the Western mental health framework slot the psychological impact of Israeli's airstrikes on Palestinian refugee camps, which have killed hundreds?

A: Individual trauma pertains to personal experiences, while collective trauma involves shared experiences of a community or group. The Western mental health framework may not fully address collective

---

* In a letter to the *Lancet*, Dr Jabr and Elizabeth Berger of the USA–Palestine Mental Health Network added: "The constant bombardment makes it impossible to find a safe place anywhere and the lack of food, water, fuel and electricity precludes the meeting of basic human needs. The once-functional mental health system has thus in the past weeks experienced a progressive shrinking of services to the degree that of six public community mental health centres, the lone remaining centre in the south has now closed and has run out of medications . . . our professional staff, accustomed to the constricted circumstances of the long-standing siege, have now experienced far deeper trauma; therapists often possess nothing but the clothes on their backs and must frequently relocate from one house to another. We must face the reality that we will be unable to rely on local capacity-building to fulfil the psychological needs of the community in Gaza."

trauma, particularly in contexts of systemic violence, displacement or dispossession, experienced by entire communities. In the Palestinian context, I see many people affected by the killing of their neighbor or classmate. I currently work with Palestinians from Jerusalem and the West Bank, who are affected by witnessing what happens in Gaza. People usually come complaining of depression, panic attacks, or anxiety. When we start talking to them and asking about their life story, then the story of grieving for someone comes up.

Q: A dehumanizing narrative accompanies the present war— some Israeli content makers are making TikTok videos mocking Palestinians' cries of suffering. World leaders have compared them to 'dogs'. Does this language distort, or normalize, people's justified misery?

A: Dehumanizing practices such as humiliation, violation of dignity and autonomy, and forced nudity, when imposed on Palestinians in various contexts, particularly in detention, arrest or during military operations, have severe and lasting effects, both psychologically and socially. These actions are not only degrading but also violate human rights, exacerbating the trauma experienced by individuals and communities. It can induce severe anxiety, depression and long-lasting psychological distress among victims.

Stripping individuals of their clothing is a direct attack on personal dignity and autonomy. It serves to humiliate and debase individuals, stripping them of their humanity, and often occurs in public or in front of others or cameras, amplifying the humiliation. Forced nudity can deeply affect an individual's sense of identity, self-worth and personal integrity. It can lead to a profound loss of self-esteem and self-respect, contributing to long-term psychological scars. Victims of forced nudity often face societal stigma and shame within their communities due to the humiliation they endured. This stigma can further isolate and marginalize individuals, impacting their relationships and social integration. It can also instil a persistent sense of vulnerability and fear in individuals; their perceptions of safety, particularly in interactions with authorities or in similar contexts, are compromized. In the long run, it can impair recovery and healing.

Q: Frank Chikane in 1986 used the term continuous traumatic stress (CTS) to explain how South Africa's Apartheid state impacted children's mental health. Can you tell us more about CTS?

A: CTS, similar to PTSD, refers to ongoing, chronic stress due to prolonged exposure to traumatic events. It can manifest in various ways and might be a more suitable framework to understand intergenerational, colonial and continued violence's psychological impact. CST finds some place in Palestinian literature, but mental health in Palestine is more layered. There are intricate historical and collective aspects here, in addition to the prolonged and repetitive nature of violence.

Q: Political philosopher Frantz Fanon argued that we cannot understand psychological problems without understanding the conditions of oppression that lead to them. Why is it important to distinguish between an individual and collective injury?

A: Distinguishing between individual and collective injury understands the broader societal impact of trauma and addresses systemic causes, rather than pathologizing individuals. Recognizing and addressing these multifaceted impacts is crucial in providing individuals and communities with adequate support and interventions.

Q: The 'We Are All Mary' campaign powerfully conveyed the experiences of Palestinian women living under oppression, while also working to heal "injuries to Palestine's social fabric", you noted. What are some conceptions of trauma that can confront intergenerational, enduring damage?

A: Palestinian culture has its own healing practices and community-based interventions that may not align with conventional Western therapeutic approaches. These could involve religious and nationalistic beliefs, storytelling, glorification of Martyrs, connection to the land (for instance, olive harvesting is like a feast for Palestinians) or community gatherings, which are deeply rooted in the cultural fabric. These practices might not be recognized or integrated into Western mental health frameworks.

Practicioners can focus on *Sumud* (steadfastness), solidarity, redress, resistance, accountability, narratives, storytelling, and community healing, contributing to addressing collective trauma beyond clinical definitions. Such efforts aim to rebuild social fabric, validate experiences, and promote resilience.

In the end, addressing collective trauma requires comprehensive approaches that go beyond clinical models. They need to embrace cultural, historical and communal healing practices—while acknowledging the systemic injustices of perpetuating suffering. We have to empower the Palestinian community to address mental health as a form of resistance against the impact of the occupation on our minds.

Mental Health Under Occupation

The Occupation in my Office: Speaking sense to power in therapeutic work

Originally published on *Middle East Eye*, 3 June 2019

Many of those ushered to my psychiatric clinic have been gripped by the crushing fist of the Israeli occupation. Others just don't fit in.

When I chose to specialize in psychiatry, a friendly colleague drew a cartoon of "Dr Samah Jabr's Clinic". The picture showed a spiderweb on the office door, implying that no one would ever come through it for psychiatric help.

He was so wrong! When I started practicing, I was surprised by the spectrum of clinical problems that people brought, often medical complaints for which doctors could find no cause. People also came for help with mood changes that affected relationships and functioning, while others sought help with bizarre, disorganized behaviour, for which traditional healers had found no explanation or treatment.

'I had become delirious'

I have also treated many individuals referred to me because they failed to fit societal expectations, including a woman who had a love affair out of wedlock, a man who did not want to get married or raise a family, a boy who was not "obedient" at school, and an adolescent wanting to change his religion. I was expected to diagnose these individuals and help them to "fit in".

Many others ushered to my clinic have been gripped by the crushing fist of the Israeli occupation. Sometimes, this presents directly, when patients arrive late with a broken leg, or don't come at all because they have been stalled at a checkpoint, beaten or arrested.

Misplaced "professional authority" can be an accomplice to oppressive power

Other times, the occupation makes its presence known indirectly, such as when a patient warned me: "Don't write my real name in your file—you are a famous doctor and the Israelis must have taken an interest in the data on your computer." This patient was not psychotic, and his concerns were not "paranoid delusions".

The occupation might also present itself unmasked, with all of its ugliness, as when a young activist told me: "I was willing to sign anything, even if they wanted me to admit that I poisoned Arafat. I just wanted to stop the endless torture and the excruciating pain; I had become delirious from sleep deprivation."

Similarly, an elderly man came to my office with suicidal ideation, which he had developed after he was forced to demolish—with his own hands—the home he had built 20 years earlier.

The hidden occupation

More often, I meet the occupation hiding within a long narrative, behind the chief complaint. I identify this hidden occupation if I'm patient enough to wait for trust to be established, and for the full story to emerge.

A woman came to see me for symptoms of anxiety that had been progressively increasing. Over a series of sessions, as she developed trust in me, she began to reveal the real cause of her symptoms: "I have told you about my husband, who has been in prison for 13 years. He will be liberated in a few months. Everyone is overjoyed to see his liberation, but I cannot share this joy. He is a stranger to me. So much has happened over the past 13 years; we are no longer the same people who once loved each other long ago."

A 47-year-old father came to see me for depressive symptoms that had prevented him from working. He denied any previous episodes, and was not interested in talking with me, wanting only a medication that would make it possible for him to return to work.

In time, however, his wife revealed what was causing her husband's depression. Their 17-year-old son had told his father, "You are not a man," when the father tried to prevent the youth from bullying his younger brother. "Where was your manhood when the soldiers came to arrest me?" the son taunted his father.

Making informed choices

No one is exempt from the burdens of the occupation. "I have no more desire for him," a rich, beautiful, lofty, middle-aged woman cried out about her husband. "Imagine, doctor, he wants to put our children in public governmental schools. My life with him has become unbearable since he lost his job." This man had been unemployed since USAID aid was cut as part of the political pressure exerted on Palestinians.

As a psychiatrist, I have the power to side with power, to give diagnoses, and to medicate. If necessary, I can write a report to hinder or exempt people from legal responsibility.

Many times, I must summarize a patient's complex story into the simple code of the International Classification of Diseases, because the establishment understands only the code. But I take the risk to speak sense to power.

My clinical encounters help me to understand how oppression operates in the mental health of people. Every day, I see how misplaced "professional authority" can be an accomplice with oppressive power, and play a role in exacerbating the suffering of individuals by telling people that their problems are only in their heads.

Not everyone who comes to see me is a "patient". Not every pain or complaint is a "symptom". Not every "fit" is a disorder.

I try to help people make sense of their painful experiences by creating an explanatory, validating narrative that gathers the complexity of their situation and negotiates their conflict with oppressive powers, rather than labeling them with a diagnostic code. I try to help them explore the battlefield that is their reality, before they make an informed choice within their own struggle to speak sense to power.

What Palestinians Experience Goes Beyond the PTSD Label

Originally published on *Middle East Eye*, 7 February 2019

In Palestine, traumatic threats are ongoing and enduring, with no "post-traumatic" safety

Elderly people in Palestine remember, with a sense of irony, the charitable parcels of clothing they received when they became refugees in 1948, as well-intentioned Westerners sent neckties, short trousers and berets to dress a population that had previously worn traditional Palestinian outfits. The new Western garments suddenly appeared on the backs of the local populace, with distinctly amusing results.

This is how the Palestinian experience of psychological morbidity looks when it is forced into ready-to-wear Western categories, such as post-traumatic stress disorder (PTSD)—the most commonly reported psychiatric disorder among Palestinians.

Journalists are fond of reporting on a high prevalence of mental health problems in Palestine to dramatize the impacts of our political reality, sometimes over-generalizing a study with limited scope so that it appears to apply to the entire population. Other times, they misinterpret epidemiological data or fail to differentiate between a symptom and a full diagnosis

Collective historical trauma

Non-governmental organizations also like the term PTSD, as it seems to help generate funds. Watching these NGOs pass out inventories of post-traumatic stress symptoms with one hand and offer food with the other, some may be tempted to express their hunger, misery and poverty by checking boxes on the survey.

PTSD is a concept developed in the context of warfare to describe the soldier's experience; it has evolved through terms such as "combat neurosis", "shell shock" and "battle fatigue", having been initially defined to account for the responses of veterans returning from Vietnam. The concept has since been broadened to include a wider range of traumatic events, including sexual violence, but it still fails to capture the experiences of communities living with collective historical trauma.

The psychiatric definition of trauma does not accommodate the most commonplace experience for Palestinians: humiliation, objectification, forced helplessness, and daily exposure to toxic stress. A child who came out of an Israeli prison claiming that the soldier who gave him a cigarette to smoke is better than his father, who denied him cigarettes, might not register PTSD symptoms on a trauma checklist, but one can suspect serious damage nonetheless.

A man who was slapped on the face, laughed at and spat upon might not have experienced "trauma" in psychiatric terms; worse still, his injury might be labelled an "adjustment disorder".

In Palestine, traumatic threats are ongoing and enduring. There is no "post-traumatic" safety. The phenomena of avoidance and hyper-vigilance are considered to be dysfunctional psychological reactions in a soldier who has returned to the safety of his hometown. But for tortured Palestinian prisoners, such symptoms are reasonable reactions, insofar as the threat lives on; they may be re-arrested and tortured again at any time.

My body is intoxicated

Western tools and instruments used in PTSD research in Palestine are not clinically or culturally validated. They do not take into consideration common Palestinian expressions of suffering. "*Badany Masmoum, Maqhour, Mazloum, Maksour Khatry*"—such are the expressions I hear most often from my patients when I ask about their feelings. These words are best translated as: "I feel that my body is intoxicated, oppressed, exposed to injustice; my desire is broken."

The well-known psychometric instruments, however, do not account for such feelings. Especially lacking is the understanding that the multiple traumas inflicted upon Palestinians due to political violence also represent a collective trauma experienced by society as a whole. As an individual trauma harms the brain tissue of a person, a collective trauma harms the integrity of the social fabric—its capacity to provide collective connections, trust, norms, world views and moral conventions.

We understand to a degree the feelings of mistrust and alienation felt by oppressed societies, but the individualized model of PTSD ignores the collective aspects of the psychological experience of Palestinians. How can we measure the psychological impact of events not aimed at individuals, such as Israel's new nation-state law, the Judaisation of Jerusalem, or the siege of Gaza?

Why is this distinction important? At the level of clinical work with individual patients in Palestine, we know what to do with our few professionals and tiny resources. We adopt and adapt to Palestinian culture, and train less-specialized people to provide low-intensity interventions in primary healthcare and school settings. Just as we build capacity for good therapists who can help traumatized individuals make sense of their experiences, we need community leaders to help the Palestinian narrative emerge in a meaningful way—to heal the collective injury.

Remembrance and reconciliation

Collective trauma can be alleviated by promoting cohesive and collective efforts, such as recognition, remembrance, reconciliation, respect for minorities, support for the afflicted, and mass cooperative action. The "We Are All Mary" solidarity campaign with Jerusalemite women, and reconciliation between aggrieved Gaza families whose children fought during the 2007 internal conflict, are examples of efforts to heal injuries to Palestine's social fabric.

The truth is that we do not have comprehensive epidemiological research on mental health in Palestine. We have a long way to go before we can draw reliable conclusions about mental health in our communities. Until then, we should examine with a critical eye the results of epidemiological surveys conducted under emergency conditions.

A dimensional approach to community mental health is more appropriate than researching the individual psychopathology of people living in a pathogenic context. As author Stefan Collini noted last year: "There are things that can be measured. There are things that are worth measuring. But what can be measured is not always what is worth measuring; what gets measured may have no relationship to what we really want to know."

Palestinians need to generate knowledge from their own experience of trauma. Qualitative research can provide important insights to help refine our conceptual definitions of trauma and delineate relevant psychometric properties. We are open to equal partnerships with international researchers who want to help us share understanding from our unique experiences. There is so much to learn about in Palestine.

A Monologue With the 'Other': The inauthenticity of discourse under occupation

Originally published on *Middle East Monitor*, 8 March 2018

The occupation of Palestine has fallen into universal oblivion. In the face of this void, however, there are still Palestinians who attempt to affirm their selfhood through challenging the occupation creatively; by refusing, for example, to submit to it with either helplessness or nihilism. Personally, I found an occasion to affirm support for Palestinian human rights and liberation in response to the decision of the International Association of Relational Psychoanalysis and Psychotherapy (IARPP) to hold its 2019 annual conference in Israel; I was among those who drafted the original letter to the IARPP leadership, calling for them to reconsider the location of the conference.

IARPP responded by refusing to reconsider the decision: "If we chose our conference locations by judging the political decisions of national governments, we might well have a hard time finding an ideal setting that would fit everyone's preferences and values." This reply, by treating Israel like any other controversial government, ignores the impact of the occupation on the possible participation in the conference itself by Palestinians and others. Placing the convenience of the conference for Israeli participants over the rights of clinicians elsewhere to have fair access to it, the organizers went on to state, "We will be extending invitations to Palestinian colleagues, and we will work to enable their presence with us. Rather than foreclosing those issues and silencing conversation, we aim to create within our relational psychoanalytic conference an open and safe space in which attendees across the political spectrum can engage and exchange views."

Apparently, the dirty work of sending colleagues who are critical of the Israeli government to airport detention centres and refusing them entry to Israel is delegated to the Israeli security forces, who in this way deny to international IARPP members the opportunity to attend the conference if they are activists within a long list of non-violent organisations, such as Jewish Voice for Peace or the American Friends Service Committee. What kind of "safe space" can thus be achieved for the exchange of diverse views at this conference can only be imagined.

This disingenuous invitation purports to display the IARPP's inclusiveness and deny culpability for its subtle support for the Israeli occupation of Palestine. The invitation also assumes the superiority of Israeli colleagues who inhabit the powerful position to "extend an invitation" to denizens of an oppressed territory. The promise of the IARPP leadership in Israel to "work to enable their presence" implies that the Israeli leadership is most generous and humane, and that Palestinians who might refuse this gracious offer simply lack gratitude. In various communications, the IARPP leadership took ownership of the virtuous language of "dialogue", the "third" and "empathy" while asserting that Palestinians who decline their kind invitation might be indulging in the reprehensible language of "splitting", "non-inclusiveness" or "acting out".

It is likely that some Palestinians will accept the Israelis' invitation, grateful for a conference hotel with close access to the Mediterranean Sea and tasty catering; they are likely to be the "good Palestinians" who accept Israeli mental health colleagues as their "professors" and do not challenge any of their reflections.

Meanwhile, to inflate the apparent Palestinian presence at gatherings of mental health clinicians, I note that the Israelis have invited pharmacists and dentists to what are professional meetings. It is more than likely that many Palestinian participants at the IARPP conference will be so impressed with the theory and jargon of relational psychology floating above their heads that they will not dare to introduce to such a group their reflections on genuinely lived Palestinian experience. We might even see the appointment of a suitably subservient Palestinian chaperone to manage the potential outbreak of genuine Palestinian discourse and to guarantee that domesticated Palestinian participants mistrust their own experience and feel ashamed of it. A nod to alleged Palestinian topics such as the problem of "Palestinians tortured by other Palestinians", or "the oppression of women under Palestinian patriarchy" might be anticipated at such an event, leaving little room to discuss or to analyze the widespread torture of Palestinians by Israelis and their overall oppression of Palestinians under occupation.

While ensuring the docility of Palestinians, the Israelis remain intimidated by critical voices among Jewish Israeli citizens and, indeed, Jews from overseas. This is yet another tactic used to silence opposition to the occupation.

Through such techniques, the Israeli pretence of dialogue remains, in fact, a monologue. The permitted voice is the mainstream Israeli view, which at most criticizes the official government view of its excesses while fundamentally endorsing the status quo. The "Other" within this masquerade is intimidated and insecure; its only permitted role is to approve the Israeli narrative with a dumb nod of the head. To fail to approve the Israeli narrative is to be the subject of spying, distorted misrepresentation and the incitement of right-wing crowds to serve as an example of the feared consequences of speaking out. In this way, others are intimidated into silence as well.

"In a narrow sense, we are not a political organisation," claims the IARPP leadership, giving them the luxury of distancing their psychological experience from the occupation while at the same time consuming the privileges of the occupation. For Palestinians, there is no such luxury; the occupation that deprives us of our loved ones, spies on our private relationships, strips our clothes from us, steals years from our lives, deprives us of our health and confronts us with continuous grief and humiliation, this is in every sense very personal and very psychological. Only those who side with the powerful are keen to ignore the dialectical relationship between the psychological and political.

The IARPP is losing a unique opportunity to respond to the voices that ask for a genuinely safe space for Palestinians and their supporters. We have had enough Israeli monologues with Palestinian "Others" who are merely decorative objects or sad examples of outright dishonesty. We need conditions in which Palestinians can bring their full authentic selves and share their true reflections. Only then can trust be established; only then can our real relationships and motivations be understood. In that safe space, we can all contribute meaningfully to political and psychological transformation that will bring a mutual emancipation and humanization for both Israelis and Palestinians.

Transcending the Borders of the Occupation

Originally published on *The Palestinian Information Center*, 13 September 2017

In a psychotic state, a 16-year-old woman patient from the West Bank went beyond the confines of her own boundaries: "I saw the sky turned red in color and I perceived a calling . . . I looked into people's eyes to see that they too were excited and understood the call of the sky."

She grasped that Jerusalem had been liberated and that she was being called to walk in its direction. Her wish for freedom and her deep desire to merge with a liberated Jerusalem, surfaced to falsify the political reality. This beautiful psychotic vision resulted in border police attacking and capturing her. Although dozens of other Palestinian youngsters have been killed at checkpoints she survived to tell her story.

Unlike the weakened psychic boundaries of my patient the geo-political boundaries and borders erected by the Israeli occupation are rigidly evident. The checkpoints not only rob us of land and natural resources—classifying and fragmenting our Palestinian identity as Jerusalemites West Bankers Gazans Palestinians of 1948 refugees and exiled individuals—but also continue to forge new identities that affirm the privilege of the occupiers and deny us our rights and integrity. Checkpoints define walls of exclusion and control and crossroads of colorful humiliation and black death for anyone who risks to "invading" the borders of her/his narrow community prison. These concrete structures have created finite parameters for our emotions, relationships, hopes, dreams, and ambitions. Damned are those who defy their borders and dare to expand their love relatedness study or work outside their cages.

Once, after giving a talk in Brussels, I was stopped by a very young Palestinian youth from Gaza. His wants were pragmatic: to help him obtain papers testifying that he is a Palestinian. This young man had become intolerant of life in Gaza and had escaped through the tunnels, enduring terrifying journeys through Egypt and several European countries before reaching Brussels. He had sacrificed all of his money and paid whatever can be paid to smugglers and dealers. When the boat carrying him arrived on the shores of Italy it sank and several of his companions died. He lost his belongings in the sea, including his identity papers and birth certificate.

In Gaza, borders have become a noose strangling the life out of its people. The siege constricts human potential by obstructing electrical work and studies and denying medical care. Recently, the Palestinian Centre for Policy and Survey Research (PSR) in the West Bank and the Gaza Strip revealed that half of the Palestinians in Gaza report that they are considering emigrating. Those who refuse to accept the slow suffocation in the besieged enclave risk their lives on an illegal boat to Europe; sadly many of them drown. The keys locking borders are used to promote dependency on the abuser. Who may cross is determined by blackmail and exploitation; there are multiple reports from patients from Gaza who were asked to be informers for the Israeli intelligence agencies in exchange for permission to cross the border to seek healthcare.

As a Palestinian Jerusalemite lacking both passport and citizenship, I am very familiar with the paradoxical feelings involved in crossing borders locally and internationally: the disgrace of being investigated as a permanent suspect; the frustration of hours and days robbed in mortifying delays; and the anxiety of not being able to cross back. And yet there is a desire to connect beyond borders the yearning to exchange knowledge and experience with the other and the aspiration to transcend the confines of the colonially imposed borders of Sykes-Picot the UN Partition Plan the Green (1949 Armistice) Line Areas A B and C, etc. I have learned many languages and the field of psychiatry as my visa and passport to symbolic border crossings into other worlds.

Working in the West Bank I cross borders every day. I experience moments of perplexity; degrading waiting and multiplicity and wealth of experience at the same time. I observe young men climbing and jumping dangerously over the eight-meter-high wall in the hope of finding work in Israeli-held areas. A few have died or been killed and many have been injured or arrested during this adventure. I observe how borders exist as concrete on the land and as thoughts in the mind. Not only are driving habits very different on the two sides of the walls but borders also make people behave and feel differently in countless ways. Between Jerusalem and the West Bank there is a gap in per capita GDP in education, health and human rights.

However, these borders do not have to be a physical wall or a checkpoint. I think of Frantz Fanon's "zones of being" and "zones of non-being", which are drawn along the virtual line that separates people according to their relative power and domination over one another.

In my land, borders are drawn with blood on the ground. They are neither natural nor neutral. They are fabricated by the Israeli occupation to maintain the power relationship between the occupiers and the natives of Palestine. Yet the fate of Palestinians should not be determined by a power relationship. Article 13 of the United Nations Declaration of Human Rights states: "Everyone lawfully within the territory of a State shall within that territory have the right to liberty of movement and freedom to choose his residence. And everyone shall be free to leave any country including his own."

While thinking of the "call" beckoning my adolescent patient to cross into Jerusalem, I look at the blue sky and I see a flock of migrant birds passing over the horizon and remember the blue sea that has swallowed many refugees and their belongings.

If there came to be justice or equality on both sides of the borders, or if there came to be respect for ethical standards or human rights within these borders and walls, then the divide between "us" and "them" would dissolve. A common pluralistic humanity would emerge around shared values and permit new middle ground and a new zone for human engagement.

Palestinian Barriers to Healing Traumatic Wounds

Originally published on *Middle East Monitor*, 20 August 2019

Traumatised patients who I see in my office often express negativistic mistrust when I ask them about their feelings: "It is humiliating to complain to anyone other than God"; "Don't complain about injuries, don't hurt anyone but yourself"; "Contain your pain in your aching heart to avoid the shame of sharing it". Such reactions are not just limited to individuals. Attitudes like these have become generalised over generations in Palestine, forming a body of maxims and proverbs that communicate a loss of faith in human relationships, a pervasive fear of danger, and an avoidance of disclosure. These reactions are barriers to healing.

The most prevalent trauma in Palestine is man-made and deliberate. What's more, the perpetrator is never held accountable, which doubles the effect of the injury. Indeed, the perpetrator enjoys impunity and inflicts guilt on its victims for the trauma itself. Guilt and shame make it difficult for people to complain or demand redress. A woman who was sexually harassed in detention gave me this reply when I proposed that she should file a report about it: "But nothing will happen if I complain! No one will believe me; the perpetrator will be defended by everyone and emerge triumphant. I will be publicly humiliated and become an object of gossip and scorn."

Political trauma in Palestine is both trans-generational and collective, and our current capacity to treat it is very limited. We lack the funding, professional resources and clinical evidence-base to address it comprehensively. Most therapies rely on treating individuals one by one and deal mainly with the here and now.

Because trauma in Palestine is so prevalent, there are overlapping ripples of traumatic grief. A young man is affected by expanding circles of injury: he lives in a refugee camp because his grandfather's home and land were seized; his mother has been preoccupied with chronic depression for 20 years following the arrest and torture of his older brother; his neighbour's home was recently demolished; his classmate was killed in a demonstration.

With this background, how do we locate the source of his chest pain when medical causes have been ruled out? The over-abundance of traumatic events in the environment make it difficult to establish aetiology; the repetition of trauma is a challenge to treatment efforts.

An additional barrier to healing is the lack of social acknowledgement of the trauma, so that isolated survivors are discouraged from seeking help. Freedom fighters who are killed in a violent context are often called terrorists by the Israeli media; to make up for this denial, Palestinian society often glorifies its political prisoners and martyrs. In this context, though, trauma victims who have been damaged by the Palestinian political system as members of an opposition group find it more difficult to recover. I have written previously about a woman who described herself as "dancing like a slaughtered chicken" after her son was killed. She feared that if she disclosed to me that he had been an Israeli informant I would become unable to empathize with her and would perceive her efforts to seek help as illegitimate. Although this was an in-depth treatment, she was profoundly avoidant of revealing the full history. She kept many parts of her trauma story ambiguous and secretive, and thus walled off from recognition and naming.

There is no safe place in Palestine. As a result, paranoia is pervasive. The lack of trust in other people is, in fact, often an appropriate safety measure rather than a psychotic symptom. When detained, prisoners are frequently told that a close friend or a relative has informed about them; others see their comrades testify against them in court. The medical field is especially suspect and my patients suspect that their psychiatric files could be used against them. Patients in Jerusalem often ask me whether my computer is connected to the Israeli national medical system. People fear that their mobile phones and computers are spying on them.

Moreover, everyday life is full of reminders of trauma. I know trauma survivors who circumscribe life into very limited spheres to avoid triggers; moving only within a small neighbourhood, for example, and losing their jobs to avoid crossing checkpoints, or ceasing to use television and social media to avoid images of soldiers' aggression. These reactions are also responses to the surrounding oppressive conditions, in which even the symbolic expression of a traumatic reality has been forbidden. People have been detained for participating in theatre, writing poetry and commenting on Facebook. These oppressive practices help us to understand why some victims of trauma are driven to repetition through re-enactment of the traumatic event.

Survivor guilt is another element complicating the recovery from trauma. I treated a teenage boy who attempted suicide several times after his cousin was killed. I later learned that this boy had encouraged his cousin to participate in political demonstrations before he was shot dead. Feelings of guilt are an important component of trauma reaction in our political context: detained women feel guilty about "leaving" their children and home; fathers of minor prisoners feel guilty about "failing" to protect them; prisoners feel guilty about "making" their parents turn their life savings over to lawyers in the hope of receiving a reduced sentence. Guilt feelings are injected regularly into people under torture when they are told things like, "We will bring your mother, wife and sisters here too" and "We will demolish your house". In many of the interactions with the oppressive Israeli administrative system, people are considered responsible for the punishment that is imposed on them; for example, homes are demolished because people "fail" to obtain the appropriate (and typically unobtainable) licence.

Palestinian dependency on Israel is another barrier to the treatment of trauma through fostering a regressive identification with the aggressor as a superior group. This dynamic adds insult to injury. A Palestinian seeking state-of-the-art therapy for a critical medical condition must travel to an Israeli hospital. A Palestinian seeking redress for torture must rely on an Israeli lawyer. When a story is told by an Israeli journalist, the narrative is perceived as more valid and credible than when it is reported by the Palestinian media. The sequestering of authority and expertise among Israelis creates further confusion in the minds of many Palestinian victims of trauma.

The lack of trust in Palestinian capacities and the ongoing narratives of nepotism, treachery, disorganization and corruption within Palestinian agencies and institutions are partially legacies of the traumatic effects of the Israeli occupation. Trauma spills over across multiple aspects of life, with an impact on social and cultural traditions, affecting the entire population, impairing critical thinking, destroying self-confidence and relationships, undermining the sense of community integrity and obscuring our hope in the future. Trauma is formative in and distorts the process of child development, the personality, interpersonal relationships, self-concept, social values and overall outlook on life.

It is comforting to have faith in the ultimate forces of fairness. However, such a belief can be dangerous for traumatized societies because it also implies that people get what they deserve. Traumatized people conclude readily that dreadful things have happened to them because they are flawed. They are convinced easily that they are essentially bad and deserve no better; their actions and behaviour will match such a conviction.

The therapist in Palestine is not immune to these pressures, and is sometimes not prepared emotionally for the challenges of trauma processing; the overwhelmed clinician is in danger of joining unwittingly with the patient's avoidance of memory and disclosure. The therapist who is not ready to ask, listen or see must work through his or her own inner barriers; he or she may be practicing a personal avoidance of trauma in unconscious collusion with the patient's resistance.

Our work in treating individual trauma wrought by political violence is part of a longer journey of healing that is faced by the entire Palestinian community. We must recover from trauma by regaining our lost normalcy through social and cultural systems that have been lingering dormant under occupation for generations. This work cannot be achieved fully in clinical office practice alone, but rather requires broad collective renewal of psychological life under conditions of autonomous agency and justice.

Permissible Pain: How to deal with traumatic images coming from Palestine

Originally published on *Middle East Monitor*, 24 May 2021

Every aggression waged by the Israeli war machine against the Palestinian people is supported by international mainstream media platforms that falsify facts and justify Israel's "right to defend itself". In reaction, local media distributes images of bleeding, maimed and shell-shocked Palestinians emerging from the rubble caused by Israeli bombardment.

These images are generated to provide evidence of the historical injustice done to our people—and sometimes, also, due to an opportunistic desire on the part of the press to provide thrills and to obtain more "likes" and "shares" on social media platforms.

As a result, we see wide-spread distribution of shocking content and images of shattered people grieving as the bodies of their loved ones are lifted out of their ruins. Some of these media intrusions dare to invade children's privacy and photograph them without their permission, with little considerations for their psychological state and the impact this image may have upon the child in the future.

I would like to mention as well the following important points, because they are often overlooked:

- The publication of these pictures of pain violates the privacy and dignity of the subjects and their families, insofar as persons in a state of shock, distress, panic and pain are not able to grant or withhold informed consent to be photographed or to have such photographs publicized.

- The distribution of images of blood, body parts and humiliating treatment competes in our memory with the beautiful images we would like to preserve of our loved ones. Instead of treasuring in our mind's eye the reassuring smile and the elegant clothes in which we usually dress ourselves for photographs, we are haunted by the most painful images of our loved ones for years after their loss. This complicates the processes of mourning and healing for their traumatic death.

- The spread of these images among the Palestinian people during times of war creates terror among those still enduring bombardment and exposed to other types of aggression. This contributes to the damage to public morale; it supports the systematic psychological warfare being waged against civilians to terrorize us and to break our will.

- Let us remember that among us there are a great many individuals from past generations who were previously traumatized by war and experienced vast circles of loss. The distribution of traumatizing images of war and devastation triggers the wounds of those formerly afflicted—as if they were experiencing the event personally in the here and now.

- Sometimes there are even worse psychological consequences to the traumatizing media content, such as the development of apathy and emotional numbness in the face of the blood and pain emanating from these images. In this way, such images lose their ability to produce any human reaction from their viewers, who calmly eat pizza while watching these images on TV.

- It is worth noting that the presence of cameras may cause people to mask their genuine feelings in an effort to maintain emotional restraint before a public audience. We see a woman holding back her tears despite her loss, trying to send her viewers a message of pride and fortitude.

- It is apparent that the official regimes in the Western world who control world politics and are complicit in the Israeli settler colonial project are not affected by images of our trauma, rather they find these images pathetic efforts to beg for sympathy. Those in the world who are in solidarity with our cause do not need heartbreaking images in order to support us; they build their solidarity on their knowledge of history, the Palestinian narrative and the facts on the ground.

- Palestinians need the solidarity of others who recognize us as active subjects and fighters for freedom, not as bleeding victims.

My call to the "camera people" is to urge them to be responsible in the face of Palestinian blood and pain. I ask them to try to convey the facts in a way that honours Palestinian sacrifices and does justice to us as Palestinians—whether as photographic subjects or as viewers.

My call to the public is to refrain from publishing traumatizing media content disrespectful of human dignity and well-being, and to withhold it from further distribution.

Leave the Judgment to God:
The role of Islamic discourse
in addressing suicide

Originally published on *Middle East Monitor*, 21 November 2019

A mother came to me in the wake of her son's suicide. She had consulted a Sheikh—in this case someone who claimed to be a religious leader—for consolation, but was told that whoever purposely kills himself will dwell in the Hellfire forever. The mother, deeply shocked, then fell into a severe depression.

It was recently reported that the Imam in a Palestinian village refused to pray for a young man who had committed suicide and delayed his burial until a few enlightened villagers took it upon themselves to bury the young man themselves. It is easy to imagine how the Imam's attitude affected the family of the deceased.

We also hear occasional reports about people with psychiatric symptoms who have sought treatment from "religious leaders"—imposters who may beat the person to "drive out the Jinn" and delay appropriate medical treatment to such a point that some persons have actually committed suicide.

I am not arguing that suicide should be permitted in a religious context. On the contrary, I believe that the prohibition of suicide is an excellent social policy for public health. I see very sick people in my clinic every day who refrain from suicide for divine prohibition.

It is the vilification of the person who has committed suicide that I oppose.

The ostracism that falls upon those who commit suicide brings shame on the surviving family members that only compounds their pain and allows the suicidal thoughts of some people to grow in silence. We should note that Islamic scholars advise that people who suffer are exonerated from obligations incumbent on the healthy and that persons who commit suicide are entitled to all the religious practices of Muslim burial.

Suicide: a medical view

While the World Health Organisation (WHO) indicates that nearly 800,000 people worldwide take their own lives, documentation of suicide in Muslim countries is generally very poor. In Palestine, statistics suggest that the number of suicides is increasing every year—but not all suicides or attempted suicides are recorded. Cases of violent death through car accidents, drug overdoses, and certain nihilistic acts of "resistance" to the occupation can be motivated by suicidal ideation—and we lack reliable records for such cases.

One of the most important risk factors for suicide is the presence of mental illness, especially depression. The risk increases when people feel that their lives are meaningless. Aggravating factors include a lack of insight, impaired judgment, disorientation, misperceptions of reality, delusions, hallucinations, medical illness and misuse of drugs or alcohol. And perhaps the most recognisable risk factor is a history of previous attempts of suicide.

The presence of family disputes, lack of social support, loneliness, financial hardship, and the spread of oppression, trauma and grief also make the decision to take one's own life more likely.

In Palestine, sadly, we lack specialized hotlines that would provide an important means to prevent suicide—and also offer an opportunity for data collection to guide research on the development of better treatment strategies.

Religiously informed medical discourse

The French sociologist Emile Durkheim emphasized the role of religion in enhancing the ability to endure suffering. Discussing the reason why suicides have been rare in Islamic societies in the past, he quoted from the Qur'an: "We estimated death among you, hastened it for some and delayed for others", concluding that nothing is more contrary to the general spirit of Islamic culture than suicide.

Olfa Mandhouj, a professor of psychology at the University of Geneva, explains that "in cases of suicide, religion should be part of the treatment," because religion deals with moral issues and the meaning of life and death. It also provides people with hope, in contrast with the feeling of emptiness experienced by most people who struggle with suicidal ideation. Indeed, having faith in great power and great meaning tends to make a person's personal problems appear less daunting.

Medically enlightened religious discourse

Most people considering suicide manage to survive by receiving support from family, friends and professionals. In Palestine, where people trust Imams and the clergy, religious counseling can be an important pillar for individuals at risk of suicide and can also play a key role in removing stigma and providing support for traumatized family members. In our society, many people suffering from psychological pain may turn to a Sheikh, or a woman preacher.

It is important to recognize that the only way to know if someone is considering suicide is to ask. Contrary to pervasive beliefs, asking about suicide will not sow the idea in a person's head and will not spread contagiously to the person who asks about it. On the contrary, directly asking about feelings provides comfort, demonstrating that the person asking has noticed something is wrong and is listening with interest; it shows that the person asked is not alone.

It is also important that persons who are not mental health professionals, including religious figures, do not make the erroneous assumption that individuals who consider suicide will improve without help. Spending time with them may save their life. Listening to what is on their minds and giving them the opportunity to speak is far more useful than sermons and intimidation.

Family and religious persons should not agree to keep a person's suicidal plans confidential. Safety must be the paramount concern. If in doubt, one should contact the person's family or friends to ensure that such persons receive appropriate help from clinical specialists. Make sure that the person seeking help knows that the door always remains open—since suicidal ideas will not disappear without substantial changes in personal conditions. And although persons struggling with suicidal thoughts can improve, they may re-experience thoughts of suicide from time to time. It is important that they know they can again receive attention and care from professionals, religious counselors, family and friends.

Anyone with experience knows how difficult it is to provide support to someone considering suicide, especially over a long period of time. It is therefore essential for specialists to train religious counselors, provide them with supervision and support them so they may be effective in providing aid, and also to protect them psychologically from vicarious trauma.

Looking forward

Studies have concluded that religious discourse based on reassurance relieves depression and anxiety, facilitates healing and promotes suicide prevention by raising morale and enhancing hope.

At the Ministry of Health, we are leading a national effort to create a comprehensive strategy for the prevention of suicide, actively seeking to upgrade suicide prevention policies by spreading community awareness and networking with the entire spectrum of service providers among the ministries and institutions within civil society, including clergy and religious institutions.

We believe that Imams and clergy are crucial partners in this effort as they are widely trusted, and because Islamic literature contains much wisdom about healing and hope. True religious leaders can lead the community in comforting the family of the deceased by offering condolences, adapting prayers to address the subject and counseling groups to process the negative emotions that naturally emerge in such situations.

In order for religious leaders to contribute to national efforts in the prevention of suicide, it is urgent and essential to introduce mental health and counseling courses in institutions for religious studies so that religious scholars are trained in the provision of psychological counseling, familiar with the vicissitudes of the human psyche, and capable of helping troubled individuals to face the difficulties that challenge human life.

It Wasn't Suicide

Originally published on *Alquds*, 20 May 2023

Israeli journalist Eddie Cohen is trying to ward off the responsibility of killing Sheikh Khader Adnan from the ruling authorities in his country by describing his heartbreaking death as suicide; some skeptics among our people picked up on this accusation and repeated it, perhaps to ward off the accusation of inaction.

What is known about Adnan is his speech full of hope, courage, altruism, sacrifice, and his bearing of responsibility towards the families of prisoners and martyrs. These qualities contradict risk factors and warning signs for people with suicidal tendencies. Whoever met Adnan once, respected him for life. It left a great positive impact on myself, on the "Beyond the Fronts" team, and on the viewers of the film, whose theme revolves around the resistance and steadfastness of the Palestinians. His presence in the film was on the occasion of the article I wrote, "Man does not live by bread alone." His interview was carried out in the hospital, where he was recovering after wresting his freedom from prison, thanks to his hunger strike in 2015.

Those who are not aware of the levels of psychological oppression and subjugation attempts to which the Palestinian prisoner is subjected, especially the administrative prisoner who does not know a reason or an end to his captivity, do not understand the option of hunger strike as a form of resistance and a final attempt to wrestle the jailer. Some may consider this option a form of psychological extremism, or an attempt to commit suicide. The hunger strike has been used as a tool of resistance in many historical movements and events, the most famous of which is its use by the Indian independence leader Mahatma Gandhi, who carried out several hunger strikes to express his objection to the policies of the British occupation in India, and it has also been used in recent years as a tool to demand political rights and freedoms in some countries.

Adnan was well versed in the issue of hunger strikes. I once heard him talk about the reasons that prompted him to go on strike, and how to prepare himself for the strike. He also explained how the strike constitutes a tool of pressure on Israel, embarrasses it, and exposes its arbitrariness and tyranny to the world.

Dr Lina Qassem, head of Physicians for Human Rights in the occupied Palestinian territory, who supervised Adnan's case, stated that he refused to break the strike, but agreed to be resuscitated if he lost consciousness, because he was not concerned with death, but with freedom, which was his main demand. He also insisted that pressure be taken to transfer him to a civilian hospital, which confirms that any talk of committing suicide is pure slander. Suicide is the killing of a person with intention and intent, but Adnan's intent was liberation. On the other hand, Adnan's doctor explained that we must pay attention to the hypothesis of force-feeding as one of the reasons that led to his death, especially since he explained to her on the 80th day of the strike that the doctors and jailers in the Ramla prison clinic had talked to him more than once about the option of force-feeding, which contradicts the Malta Declaration approved by the International Federation of Doctors in 1991. This clearly defines instructions for dealing with hunger strikes, indicating that force-feeding is unacceptable and absolutely unacceptable from a moral point of view.

Who is responsible? The Israeli judiciary, which delayed and procrastinated in handling his case, the Prison Authority, which failed to transfer him to the hospital so that he could be saved, and the absence of unified national support. For everyone who asks, "Did Adnan commit suicide?" the answer is: "It was not suicide, rather he was deliberately killed, and we consider him a martyr with God, and we do not commend anyone before God." Khader Adnan will remain a shining star that lights up the darkness of occupied Palestine, like Sherine Abu Aqleh and other free Palestinians.

On The Misuse Of Psychiatry In Inciting Violence Against Palestinians

Originally published on LinkedIn, January 2024

Recent statements by Ayelet Shmuel, an Israeli psychotherapist and the director of the International Resilience Center in Sderot, are deeply troubling and morally reprehensible. She "diagnoses" the entire Palestinian population as "sociopaths" and incites for their murder, claiming "soon they will have no thumbs to play with rockets." In the context of an ongoing genocide that has claimed the souls of thousands in Gaza, these remarks not only lack empathy but also perpetuate a dangerous narrative of hate and violence.

Using psychiatric classification to perpetuate racism is a dangerous and regressive path. History has shown us how such categorizations have been misused to oppress and marginalize oppressed groups. From "drapetomania," the diagnosis applied to slaves fleeing from captivity, and "dysaesthesia aethiopica," the diagnosis applied to a "lazy" slave, to, more recently, the diagnosis of "sluggish schizophrenia" characterizing dissidents in the USSR, these politically motivated examples underscore the dangerous intersection of psychiatry and prejudice.

Shmuel's rhetoric is a stark reminder of the misuse of power, the manipulation of psychiatric language to further political agendas, and the perpetuation of systemic racism. Her callous statements not only disregard the humanity of Palestinians but also echo a painful history of dehumanization used to justify violence against marginalized communities.

If Shmuel genuinely seeks to understand the dynamics of power, oppression, and sociopathy, she should turn her attention to the hundreds of documented experiences of torture inflicted by Israeli soldiers who interrogate Palestinian political detainees. Instead of promoting hatred and violence, she should engage in professional efforts aimed at documenting and addressing the psychological trauma inflicted by the occupation.

I invite Shmuel to explore the realm of anticolonial liberation psychology, which challenges oppressive power structures and highlights the ethical responsibility of a mental health professional and advocates for the emancipation of all human beings. This approach emphasizes the importance of justice, equality and genuine liberation for all, acknowledging that the liberation of one group does not come at the expense of another.

Why US Mental Health Associations Justify Israel's Genocidal Attack on Gaza

Originally published on *Middle East Eye*, 15 October 2023

One-sided condemnations from leading psychiatric associations reinforce Israeli propaganda and make them accomplices to oppression and killing of Palestinians.

This week, the American Psychiatric Association (APA) issued a statement on the "terrorist attacks in Israel" and the American Academy of Child & Adolescent Psychiatry (AACAP) released a similar response to the "recent attacks and acts of terror in Israel". As they currently stand, these are disappointingly one-sided condemnations and fail to address Israel's 75-year-long occupation of Palestine and numerous atrocities committed against Palestinians throughout this period.

While the APA portrays Palestinian resistance as antisemitism and terrorism, an occupied people's right to resist is both legal under international law and, like mental health itself, a basic human right. The appalling imbalance in the stated positions of the APA and the AACAP reflects a dangerous lack of awareness or wilful ignorance of the physical and mental health effects of the occupation, particularly the Gaza siege, on Palestinians.

By failing to address the long-term suffering of Palestinians and unequivocally siding with the occupier, the APA and AACAP have violated their own principles of impartiality and neutrality and exposed their lack of commitment to addressing the mental health needs of all people.

Unequal lives

The statements by the world's leading psychiatric associations neglect the historical context and cast a blind eye to the besieged population in Gaza, half of whom are children. They make no mention of the horrific bombardment of the tiny enclave or what many rights groups are now calling a genocide against Palestinians.

It seems obvious that mental health professionals' concerns should extend to all people equally. Who better than psychiatrists to understand the importance of freedom?

By the same token, the statements totally ignore the psychological impact and trauma of the occupation. Rights groups have documented the inhumane conditions for years, including reports by Physicians for Human Rights, Amnesty International and Save the Children, among others.

In its brutal campaign of collective punishment, Israel has cut off food, fuel, electricity, water and medical supplies, and in what is being described as a second Nakba, has displaced hundreds of thousands of Palestinians who were forced to flee their homes.

One-third of the more than 2200 Palestinians killed and the nearly 9000 injured so far in Gaza are children, yet their lives were apparently unworthy of mention by the AACAP.

Even in its half-hearted statement on the current "crisis" in Gaza, the AACAP cannot bring itself to "mourn" the children killed, expressing nothing more than a vague concern for potentially distressing "imagery" to which the children may potentially be exposed.

It is as though young teens were not forced to endure five Israeli wars on Gaza, with massive civilian death tolls, during the last decade and a half.

Beyond the horrific violence, Gaza has been depleted by a crippling 16-year blockade, described as an open-air prison with the highest population density. In the last few days, more than one million people have been ordered by Israel to leave their homes with nowhere to go.

It seems obvious that mental health professionals' concerns should extend to all people equally. Who better than psychiatrists to understand the importance of freedom for human beings—for Palestinians and Israelis alike? Otherwise, the only explanation for such clear double standards is that the APA and AAPAC have adopted wholesale the official Israeli narrative and are unable to see Palestinians as humans.

Dangerous propaganda

The statements further dehumanise Palestinians by ignoring their enduring mental health challenges and collective trauma, resulting from decades of oppression, ongoing violence, humiliation and injustice inflicted by the occupation.

The bombing of Palestinian schools, ambulances and hospitals—including the only psychiatric hospital in Gaza, which took place on Friday morning as I learned from its director and my colleague, Dr Abdullah Aljamal—is but one instance of these chronic harms.

Such statements from medical organizations, which are allegedly not a political lobby, further inflame public sentiment and reinforce dangerous propaganda supporting Israel's genocidal actions towards Palestinians in Gaza. Instead, the APA and AACAP could have done better to confront the vicious lies spread by the US government and media, including the horrific, and since debunked, "beheaded babies" smear.

If these organizations were truly concerned for the well-being of civilians or children, they could have confronted the massive arsenal of US military aid to Israel, which assists Israel in implementing its murderous plans against Palestinians.

Hubristic attitudes

The APA and AACAP would better serve the people of Israel by helping them to shed their hubristic attitudes and sense of entitlement. They could help stem future violence by recognizing the legitimate struggle of Palestinians to live in freedom and dignity and recognize that wherever there is oppression, there will be resistance.

A more balanced and empathetic approach is essential, one that acknowledges the mental health struggles on both sides and advocates for a just and peaceful resolution for both peoples. A principled resolution must be based on human rights and international law.

Mental health as a fundamental human right was the theme of the latest World Mental Health Day on 10 October. Working towards global mental health demands a comprehensive and inclusive perspective that truly supports all those impacted by this longstanding and ongoing crisis.

Palestinian psychiatrists and mental health professionals call upon all colleagues, and health and mental health organizations globally, to uphold the ethics of our professional role and not be corrupted by political ideology.

We must push back against the APA and AAPAC and any other professional organizations that contribute to hateful and negative representations of the Palestinian people. Such dangerous statements make them accomplices of the oppression and killing of Palestinians.

Killing After Killing: Genocidal tactics and Palestinian ultimate witnessing

Not published, written in July 2024

While Israel and its Western allies question the accuracy of Palestinian casualty figures and accuse the Gaza Ministry of Health of inflating the numbers, three experts from the *Lancet* medical journal published a letter on 5 July 2024 estimating that indirect deaths caused by factors such as impaired reproductive health and non-communicable diseases might mean the death toll is several times higher than official Palestinian estimates. The letter suggests it is plausible that up to 186,000 deaths could be attributed to the current situation in Gaza. The authors stated this is a conservative estimate based on trends from prior conflicts, estimating four indirect deaths for every direct death.

For decades, Palestinians have endured systematic violence, killing, destruction, and profound psychological trauma under Israeli occupation. Israel's ground and air campaign in Gaza, initiated on October 7 in response to Palestinian resistance fighters breaching Gaza's borders, has resulted in more than 38,000 deaths and displaced 2.3 million people from their homes. Regardless of the exact casualty numbers, the massive scale of killing in Gaza exemplifies the brutal reality of war, where death assumes multiple dimensions with devastating consequences. This essay explores the direct and indirect forms of killing Palestinians in Gaza, its impact on survivors, and the unique cultural perspective on martyrdom within the Palestinian community.

Direct killing through bombardment

The most immediate and visceral form of killing since October 2023 is through massive bombardment. It is estimated that the number of bombs dropped on Gaza, an area a third the size of Hiroshima, is seven times greater than those dropped on Hiroshima. This form of killing aims to shock the civilian population and intimidate neighboring countries. Such massive killing reduces human lives to mere numbers and statistics. Reports indicate that artificial intelligence has been used to determine targets, with people appearing on Israeli monitors as tiny black-and-white figures, resembling insects. Israeli pilots who execute these attacks cannot hear the cries of the dying Palestinians, highlighting the dehumanization inherent in such acts, stripping individuals of their identities and reducing them to collateral damage.

Indirect killing: starvation and health system destruction

Beyond immediate violence, the systematic destruction of essential infrastructure perpetuates killing, particularly through the health system's obliteration and weaponized starvation. The *Lancet* article underscores the extensive destruction of Gaza's health infrastructure. In June, the UN Human Rights Office reported the killing of 500 health workers in Gaza since 7 October 2023, amidst systematic attacks on medical facilities, violating the laws of war. This has created a crisis in public health and hygiene, with people dying from infected wounds and increased maternal and infant mortality.

Health workers have faced serious violations, including mass detention and enforced disappearances during Israeli raids on hospitals such as Al Awda, Kamal Adwan, Al Shifa Medical

Complex, and Al Amal hospitals. Since October 7, more than 300 health workers have been detained by the Israeli military forces, with many reporting torture and ill-treatment in custody. Some Palestinian doctors reportedly died in detention due to torture, including Dr Adnan Al Bursh, head of the orthopedic department at Al Shifa Hospital, and Dr Iyad Al Rantisi, head of the obstetrics and gynecology department at Kamal Adwan Hospital.

The killing, detention, torture, and enforced disappearance of health workers, along with the destruction of most medical facilities, have devastated Gaza's healthcare system. This collapse has exacerbated the suffering of civilians, especially with the spread of communicable diseases affecting children, older people, pregnant women, and those with disabilities.

Starvation as a weapon of war
Starvation, a slow and agonizing form of death, emerges from the blockade and destruction of food supplies. Over the past seven months, Israel has rapidly starved 2.3 million Palestinians in Gaza, leading to the first reported deaths of children by starvation in January 2024. Today, Gaza faces a famine with irreversible consequences, especially for children, whose brain development is affected by anemia and malnutrition. Even if the conflict ended now, Gaza's food systems are destroyed, with one-third of agricultural lands, the fishing fleet, and irrigation systems decimated. Starvation is being used as a weapon of war, causing genocidal violence.

Such forms of killing, through the destruction of the health system and deliberate starvation, though less visible, are equally insidious and morally reprehensible, highlighting the extended reach of war's lethal impact.

Killing after death: denying burial

The act of killing extends even beyond death. In Gaza, 30% of those counted dead in emergency rooms remain unidentified, and an estimated 10,000 bodies remain under the rubble of residential homes. The ongoing violence prevents proper burial and mourning rituals, a profound psychological weapon that denies families a normal closure of their pain. Horrible scenes of mass graves, cadavers being eaten by starving wild dogs and cats, and rotting bodies spread all over Gaza perpetuate the suffering of the living, entrenching trauma and helplessness in the community. This posthumous violence reflects a deeper psychological assault on human dignity, denying the dead their final rites and the living their peace.

Psychological killing of survivors

Survivors of Gaza genocide endure a different, yet equally harrowing, form of killing. The trauma inflicted by witnessing and experiencing extreme violence leads to profound psychological scars. People in Gaza have seen their relatives buried alive in the rubble, witnessed mass graves of blindfolded and handcuffed people, and heard of chilling accounts of torture of their relatives. Such cruelty is designed to freeze survivors in a state of perpetual terror and helplessness, leaving their lives forever altered. This psychological assassination of people's souls and spirits leaves surviving bodies as hollow shadows of their former selves, with profound trauma causing ongoing and pervasive suffering.

Existential implications

The ease of killing Palestinians raises fundamental philosophical questions about the nature of humanity and the meaning of life. The deliberate destruction of human life, whether through direct violence or indirect means, challenges our moral frameworks, social contracts, and belief in human rights and international law. The televised dehumanization of Palestinians, the reduction of their lives to mere statistics, and the prolonged suffering inflicted on survivors highlight profound moral and ethical dilemmas about the meaning of justice and human dignity.

The glorification of martyrs

At one international NGO, the administration objected to an employee's use of the term "Shaheed" while the employee, a psychologist, was telling the story of a grieving mother of a martyr. "This is not a professional term," they argued.

In oppressed communities like the Palestinians, the figure of the martyr holds profound significance. Palestinians refer to their martyrs as *Shuhada*, meaning "the ultimate witnesses." This term reflects the belief that martyrs fully see and testify to the horrors of war and injustice. They become symbols of resistance to tyranny, embodying the collective suffering and enduring spirit of their people. The use of the title "martyr" preserves their memory and honors their sacrifice, maintaining reverence and solidarity within the community. Each martyr's story becomes a testament and contribution to the ongoing struggle for Palestinian freedom and liberation.

With all due respect for international NGOs and their "professional" administration, the term *Shaheed* triggers fear and discomfort in those who seek a killing after killing for Palestinians. The glorification of martyrs by Palestinians highlights the enduring human spirit and quest for justice in the face of overwhelming killing and denial; the term summarizes Palestinian history and explains the violent oppressive context in which a Palestinian loses their life. This is a respectable way to revive lost souls, offer condolence to their families, and undo the tactics of genocide.

Occupation is a Mental Health Issue

Occupation and the Mind

Published on *New Internationalist*, 1 May 2007

Ahmad, a 46-year-old man from Ramallah, was doing well, until his last detention. But this time he just could not tolerate the long incarceration in a tiny cell, with complete visual and auditory deprivation. First, he lost his orientation to time. Then he became over-attentive to the movement of his gut and started thinking that he was "artificial inside his body." Later, he developed paranoid thinking, started hearing voices and seeing people in his isolated cell. Today, Ahmad is out of his detention, but still imprisoned by the idea that everyone is spying on him.

Fatima spent several years doctor-shopping for a combination of severe headaches, stomach aches, joint pain and various dermatological complaints. There was no evidence of an organic cause. Finally, Fatima showed up at our psychiatric clinic and spoke of how all her symptoms started after she saw the skull of her murdered son, open on the stairs of her house, during the Israeli invasion of her village of Beit Rima on 24 October 2001.

Such are the cases I see in my clinic. The traumatic events of war have always been a major source of psychological damage. In Palestine the kind of war being waged needs to be understood in order to appreciate the psychological impact on this long-occupied population. The war is chronic and continuous, over the lifetime of at least two generations. It pits an ethnically, religiously and culturally foreign state against a stateless civilian population. In addition to daily oppression and exploitation, it involves periodic military operations of usually moderate intensity. These provoke occasional Palestinian factional and individual responses. The vast majority of people are never consulted about such actions. While their opinion does not matter, it is they who must endure pre-emptive Israeli strikes or collective punishment in retaliation for acts of Palestinian resistance.

Displacement

Demographic factors complicate the picture. Those living in the occupied territories make up just a third of Palestinians; the rest are scattered around the region in a diaspora, many in refugee camps. Almost every Palestinian family has experiences of displacement or major painful separation. Even inside Palestine, people are refugees, expelled in 1948 to live in refugee camps. The massive displacement of 70% of the people, and the destruction of over 400 of their villages, are referred to by Palestinians as the Nakba or Catastrophe. This remains a trans-generational psychological trauma, scarring Palestinian collective memory. Very often, you will encounter young Palestinians who introduce themselves as residents of towns and villages their grandparents were evacuated from. These places are frequently no longer on the map, either razed entirely, or now inhabited by Israelis.

Palestinians perceive Israel's war against them as a national genocide, and to resist it they give birth to many children. The fertility rate among Palestinians is 5.8—the highest in the region. This leads to a very young population (53% under the age of 17), a vulnerable majority, at a crucial stage of physical and mental development. The geographical enclosure of Palestinians in very small neighbourhoods, with the separation wall and a system of checkpoints, encourages consanguineous marriages, increasing a genetic predisposition to mental illness. Walling off friends and neighbours from each other also has a debilitating effect on the cohesion of Palestinian society.

But it is the violent environment in which they live which most undermines the mental health of Palestinians. Population density, especially in Gaza—with 3823 persons per square kilometre—is very high. Elevated levels of poverty and unemployment—67% and 40% respectively—undermine hope and deform personality. The war has left us with a huge community of prisoners and ex-prisoners, estimated at 650,000, or some 20% of the population. The disabled and mutilated make up 6%. Recent screenings found a disturbing level of anaemia and malnutrition, especially among youngsters and women. The intense emotional hostility provoked by our daily friction with the Israeli soldiers at our doorsteps is a constant stress factor. Many Palestinian kids have been living with daily violence since birth. For them, the noise of bombardment is more familiar than the singing of birds.

Sudden blindness

During my medical school training in several Palestinian hospitals and clinics, I saw men complaining of non-specific chronic pains after they lost their jobs as labourers in Israeli areas. I also saw schoolchildren brought in for secondary bed-wetting after a horrifying night of bombardment. And all too vivid is my memory of a woman, brought to the emergency room suffering from sudden blindness that started when she saw her child murdered as a bullet entered his eye and exited from the back of his head.

In Palestine, such cases are not registered as war injuries and are not treated properly. This realization provoked me to specialize in psychiatry. It is one of the most underdeveloped medical fields in Palestine. For a population of 3.8 million, we have 15 psychiatrists and are understaffed with nurses, psychologists and social assistants. We have an estimated 3% of the staff we need. We have two psychiatric hospitals, in Bethlehem and Gaza, but it is difficult to get to them, due to checkpoints. There are seven outpatient community mental-health clinics. In developing countries like occupied Palestine, psychiatry is the most stigmatized and the least financially rewarding medical profession. Psychiatrists work with desperately sick patients and, in the eyes of their communities, are far removed from the glory of other medical specialties. As a result, competent and talented doctors rarely specialize in psychiatry.

I find psychiatry a humanizing and dignifying profession—not least because it helps me to cope with all the violence and disappointments surrounding me. I move from Ramallah to Jericho to see psychiatric patients. In one working day I see between 40 and 60 patients; 10 times the number I used to see during my training in Parisian clinics. I observe my patients' disorganized behaviour, listen to their overwhelming stories and answer them with the few means I have: a bit of talking to pull together their fragmented ideas; some pills that might help them to organize their thinking, stop their delusions and hallucinations, or allow them to sleep or calm down. But talks and pills can never return a killed child to his parents, an imprisoned father to his kids, or reconstruct a demolished home.

The ultimate solution for mental health in Palestine is in the hands of politicians, not psychiatrists. So, until they do their job, we in the health professions continue to offer symptomatic treatment and palliative therapy—and sensitize the world to what is taking place in Palestine.

Resistance

Nowadays, Palestinians are pressured to surrender once and for all, when they are asked to "recognize" Israel. We are asked to accept, reconcile ourselves with and bless the Israeli violation of our life. The fact that our homeland is occupied does not, by itself, mean that we are not free. We reject the occupation in our minds, as far as we can cope with it; and learn how to live in spite of it, rather than being adjusted to it. But if we recognize Israel, we are mentally occupied—and that, I claim, is incompatible with our well-being as individuals and a nation. Resistance to the occupation and national solidarity are very important for our psychological health. Their practice can be a protective exercise against depression and despair.

Israel has created awful facts on the ground. What remains for us of Palestine is a thought, an idea that becomes a conviction of our right to a free life and a homeland. When Palestinians are asked to "recognize" Israel, we are asked to give up that thought, and to renounce everything we have and are. This will only sink us deeper into an eternal collective depression.

After several years in Paris I returned to a tired, starved Palestinian people, torn apart by factional conflicts as well as by the separation wall. Palestinians are especially demoralized by the infighting taking place on the streets of Gaza, but orchestrated elsewhere in order to abort the results of last year's democratic elections. Those who have stopped all money from going to Palestine are, in effect, sending us guns instead of bread. They encourage the psychologically and spiritually impoverished to kill their neighbours, cousins and ex-classmates. Even if the factions settle up, Palestinian society will be left with a serious problem of intra-family revenge.

We shall overcome

It is hard not to wonder whether Israel's targeting of Palestinians is deliberately designed to create a traumatized generation; passive, confused and incapable of resistance. I know enough about oppression to diagnose the non-bleeding wounds and recognize the warning signs of psychological deformity. I worry about a community forced to extract life from death and peace through war. I worry about youth who live all their lives in inhumane conditions, and about babies who open their eyes to a world of blood and guns. I am concerned about the inevitable numbness chronic exposure to violence brings. I also fear the revenge mentality—the instinctive desire to perpetuate on your oppressors the wrongs committed against yourself.

There has yet to be a comprehensive epidemiological study of the psychological disorders in Palestine. And, despite all that is published on Palestinian war-related psychopathology, my impression is that mental illness is still the exception in Palestine. Resilience and coping are still the norm among our people. In spite of all the home demolitions and extreme poverty, it is not in Palestine you find people sleeping in the streets or eating from trash cans. This resilience is based on family foundations, social steadfastness and spiritual and ideological conviction.

Still, we do have a mental-health emergency. Services are urgently needed for people who have suffered and endured crises so that they can restore their recuperative powers and coping capacities. This is crucial if they are not to crack when peace finally comes, as so often occurs in a postwar period. It is not just a small number of sick individuals but an entire wounded society that needs care. Our trauma has been chronic and severe; but by recognizing our suffering and treating it with faith and compassion, we shall overcome.

Our History Haunts Our Future

Originally published on *Middle East Monitor*, 15 May 2018

A French colleague once asked me, "Why are the Palestinians stuck in the Nakba? They commemorate villages no longer present on any map and bequeath to their children the keys to homes that have been long abandoned. Why don't they leave it all behind, and look to the future?"

The answer is that the Nakba is not only an historical trauma but an accumulative affliction that continues to harm Palestinian identity, both collectively and individually; the Nakba is an ongoing injury that has never been bandaged or healed. The Nakba is a contemporary insult renewed with every Palestinian who is humiliated, arrested and killed; salt is added to the wound of the Nakba with every demolished home and every bit of confiscated land.

The memory of the Nakba is not kept alive by the key that moves from the hand of the grandfather to the hand of the grandson. The memory lies in the damaged identity and self-image that has been thrust upon us and which is passed from generation to generation. We inherit the Nakba from the oppressed, expelled generation which came before—an anguished heritage that carries bad memories as if our genes themselves were anguished.

Neither an attempt to forget or the senility of old age can dispel these memories. Silence cannot undo its shocking impact. On the contrary, commemoration of the Nakba is necessary in order to understand the present and to redress the injury of the past. A collective trauma requires a collective healing through popular narrative, rituals, and symbolic representation, as well as restorative justice. Silence and denial will only deepen the wound and inflict future calamities upon us.

"But the Palestinians who approach the fence in Gaza must be suicidal!" proclaims my colleague emphatically, without curiosity about the thoughts and feelings of these Palestinians. My colleague's quick diagnosis does not acknowledge that these Palestinians may intend to communicate a need, may intend to alter the unchanging conditions of the status quo. These Palestinians may intend to protest the theft of their land or the siege or the partition of their people. But by making a quick diagnosis, my colleague forecloses the opportunity to listen and to negotiate better strategies; by drawing judgments on the basis of surface behavior, genuine understanding is short-circuited.

There is a difference between the psychological profile of a person who attempts suicide because of personal problems and the person who undergoes self-sacrifice in the context of social struggle. The suicidal person is hopeless and desperate, withdrawing from others pessimistically or fearing to be a burden upon them. Suicidal actions are often egocentric because the individual's spark of life has lost its meaning in interpersonal terms. In contrast, the self-sacrificing person—even on the pathway to death—may be full of hope, indeed perhaps too much so. The act of self-sacrifice often involves an altruistic dedication to others and an eagerness to improve their future chances. Their hope is to extinguish their own soul in the service of giving light to others and brighten the road ahead.

I remember a dream I had a few years ago. I was walking in the darkness and beheld creatures with brown fur walking slowly on their four legs. Every now and then, one stopped and turned its head upwards. It was too dark to see clearly, but I finally recognized a human face. That was a dream about my people and the poor insight in the world.

When Palestinians fight for their national rights we are called "terrorists." When we demonstrate in non-violent ways and are killed by the occupying forces, we are called "suicidal;" Avi Dichter, the Chairman of the Israeli Foreign Affairs and Defense Committee, called peaceful demonstrators "idiots."

Are there people who are willing to open their eyes in this darkness to see the Palestinian human face?

Throughout history, millions have marched to have their voices heard. Human beings often make sacrifices for the sake of their values or on behalf of others for whom they care. When such persons die, they are glorified and considered to be martyrs to their cause. Why should it be so different when such persons are killed by Israeli forces? Two months ago, Arnaud Beltrame, a French policeman, exchanged himself with a hostage in a terrorist attack in Trebes; he was unfortunately killed, but his behavior was lauded as brave and heroic, not suicidal.

The great march which started on Land's Day and continues as I write this text, on the bitter occasion of the establishment of the American Embassy in my occupied city of Jerusalem, is meant to celebrate the 70th Anniversary of the Nakba. This march signifies the special meaning of this land to the Palestinians. Whereas some landowners may regard their lands as mere property that generates economic profit and can be exploited for water, energy and food, the Palestinians feel otherwise. As a landless people, the Palestinians view land as an aspect of their own souls, representing their injured identity. Attached to their land with deep emotion, many Palestinians are ready to die for it. Advocacy, strategies, planning and calculation of risks are needed so that Palestinians do not need to be killed in order for their plight to be recognized. Premature judgment, psychiatric labeling, or exploitation of self-sacrifice cannot advance understanding of this plight.

Land is the material space for the life story of Palestinians, as with all people. Let there be space on earth for the Palestinians, so that human beings will not search for their life stories underground. It is a great anguish that so many Palestinians are killed in defense of their dreams. Our only solace is to believe that if they have left us by choice to sleep forever, they continue somehow to pursue those beautiful dreams.

Talking Through Our Fears: Resisting the Palestinian complacency of silence

Originally published on *Middle East Monitor*, 11 August 2018

On a few occasions, my mother has awakened me anxiously to let me know who is the latest to be arrested for a Facebook statement, and to warn me from posting my views on my page. And when I say goodbye before my trips abroad, she responds with a warning: "Don't get involved in politics and don't say anything about Israel!" I always reply with an effort at humour, "My talk is about Palestinian mental health. Israel has nothing to do with mental health—it has to do with mental illness." But my mother doesn't relax or laugh at my attempts at reassurance. I leave quickly before I am affected by her contagious fears.

My mother is not the only one to hand over to the occupation a free service of self-censorship. There are common expressions encouraging silence in Palestine: "The walls have ears" and "Walk quietly along the wall and ask God to cover you." Yet even worse is the clergy who maintain "silence is a sign of acceptance" when confronted with a silent bride in a marriage ceremony. One does not need to be a psychiatrist to see that silence is more often a sign of intimidation and fear.

The Palestinian reality has silenced a few Palestinians forever, such as the writer Ghassan Kanafani and the cartoonist Naji Al-Ali who were killed on account of their opinions. Several others have been arrested for expressing their thoughts freely. The poet Dareen Tatour was convicted for her poem, "Resist, my people, resist them." It was judged by the Israelis as an "incitement to violence."

Yet all the while, the posts of the Israeli rapper The Shadow are not considered an "incitement to violence," although one of his posts displays him holding an image of testicles accompanied by the words: "Revenge, Bibi [the nickname of Israeli Prime Minister], I think you forgot these!" In another post, the rapper calls on the Israeli army's medical team to cut out the organs of Palestinians whom they have killed in order to donate them to the Israeli National Transplant Center. Israel is equally tolerant of the "free speech" of the authors of *The King's Torah*, who explain that the injunction "Thou Shall Not Kill" applies only to "a Jew who kills a Jew." *The King's Torah* then states that non-Jews are "uncompassionate by nature" and attacks upon them are justified because they "curb their evil inclinations." Similarly, the babies and children of Israel's enemies may be killed without compunction, since "it is clear that they will grow [up] to harm Jews."

Israelis get away with saying such things, even gaining popularity and status because of these statements. We remember in this context how Alelet Shaked as a member of the Knesset described women in Gaza as "snakes" and incited killing them during the attack of 2014. Today she is the Israeli Minister of Justice!

Recently, Lama Khater, a Palestinian journalist critical of Israel, was sent to prison in Israel—joining 22 other journalists who are likewise imprisoned. Frequently, people in Palestine are dismissed from their jobs or lose other opportunities for daring to voice political views that do not properly conform to acceptable opinions. Outside of Palestine, students whose activism focuses on Palestine are threatened in their studies and in their opportunities for employment. Even retired persons internationally who are friends of Palestine worry about the right to travel to Palestine and receive threats, such as the Jewish Brigade's menace to scalp French activists in the Association France Palestine Solidarite.

Paradoxically, while some are harmed for speaking up, others are harmed for choosing not to speak. Among my psychiatric patients in Palestine, I have seen a woman suffering from aphonia—the loss of her voice—because intelligence forces working for the Israelis blackmailed her about her socially prohibited phone calls to her lover. A young Palestinian activist with a secret homosexual relationship was threatened with being "outed from the closet", and intentionally inflicted with hemorrhoids and sexually transmitted diseases if he refused to collaborate with the Israelis. There were those who were injured but left to die in Gaza because they refused to inform on activists in exchange for permission to gain access to medical services outside of Gaza.

Working through silence is a daily activity in my work. I see many people with shortness of breath and chest pain—symptoms caused because they feel they are drowning in society. There are many people with sexual dysfunctions brought about because they cannot communicate openly about their relationship. There are victims of torture who are silent about their experience because they believe that reporting is hopeless or because they fear further revenge. There are depressed individuals who remain quiet about their suicidal thoughts because they anticipate rejection or fear being locked up in a hospital. I know the cost of silence, found in the pathology—acting out aggression or becoming dysfunctional.

Outside my clinic, I am always confronted with questions of safety regarding my public speaking: "Don't you worry about going to prison, or fear that other harms will come to you because you're speaking up and writing?" Those with less good intentions might say, "But isn't the very fact that you are here and able to speak itself evidence that Israel is a real democracy?"

I talk, not only in order to be a coherent person, both inside and outside my professional role, but because I cannot do otherwise. I cannot pretend I do not know; I cannot deny my feelings about the political reality; I cannot turn my face the other way. I speak to protest against violence and to attempt to engage in a genuine critical dialogue with the other. This is the best that I can do in the face of an oppressive reality. Expressing my thoughts is the heart-beat of my humanity. This is the most basic right, without which no other human rights can be established.

In my work, I have seen hypochondriacal patients who act as if they are sick, out of their fear of being sick. In my daily life, I encounter people who live like the poor, out of their fear of poverty. I have seen people who are not able to communicate in their relationships, out of their fear of abandonment. I do not want to waste my opportunities as these people have done and live imprisoned in my own mind out of fear of being thrown into a concrete prison. I do not deny that I have this fear, but I am trying to talk through it and in spite of it.

When Israel attacked Gaza in 2014, I initiated a petition calling professionals to stand in solidarity with Palestinians. I then discovered that the attack on Gaza left some collateral damage in my heart—once I saw that some close colleagues were unwilling to sign the petition and indeed pressured me to withdraw it. While I respect and empathize with the factors that may constrict the choices of many of the people around me, I am not by nature an impulsive, risk-taking individual. In speaking out, I calculate the necessary risks and balance these risks against the benefits of achieving wider margins for freedom of expression. I sometimes consult with Israeli lawyers to ensure that my actions are not in breach of the unjust laws governing the occupation. During the First Intifada, it was illegal to hold the Palestinian flag; nowadays, it is illegal to associate with BDS. Although these two actions are just and moral, I never held a Palestinian flag and I have not joined BDS. My aim is to create alternative forms of expression that are not in breach of unjust laws—and are probably therefore more effective strategies for me.

I have always calibrated the scope of my articulated opinions with the dimensions of my professional identity and financial autonomy. Moreover, I am careful in my risk-taking that I do not implicate others. I continue to avoid deriving my personal income from Israeli institutions and remain a public employee in the Palestinian system. Clearly, being an employee, especially a public employee, is often antagonistic with free expression and over time can pollute one's conscience and capacity to think freely. But until I am no longer employed as a public employee, I will try to maintain diversified sources of income through freelance consultations and work with more than one institution at the same time; in this way, I hope to avoid being wholly dependent upon a single employer, who can dictate my speech.

To further protect myself, I base my writings and talks on well-established facts. I share my opinions based on such facts, referring not only to Palestinian experience, but also to international human rights and universal values that are presumed to govern both Israelis and Palestinians alike. I write in foreign languages in order to recruit more witnesses to my experience. I trust that many people in solidarity will speak up on my behalf, should something bad befall me.

I am mindful as well that I have been protected by the activities of more courageous Palestinians than I, who have kept the Israelis busy with more weighty struggles than I can undertake. I count on the premise that Israeli "intelligence" that will make the judgment call that "stopping" me would be counterproductive, as it would bring more attention to the very voice that they hope to silence.

And perhaps I am simply naïve; perhaps my risk assessment is nothing more than my sophisticated denial of political threat. If that be the case, then let this article be my manifesto—a refusal to surrender the right to speak and to fall into the collective complacency of silence.

The Assassination of Palestinian Memory: Another tool of ethnic cleansing

Originally published on *Middle East Monitor*, 18 May 2019

While Israel was celebrating its independence day earlier this week, I heard two anecdotes.

One story was related to me by Jerusalemite friends working in Israeli institutions, who told me about their discomfort during Yom HaZikaron—the day of remembrance honoring Israeli soldiers who have fallen and honoring other Israelis who have died due to "terrorism." On that day in Israel, a siren is sounded across the country and all persons are expected to stop whatever they are doing—including driving an automobile—to demonstrate through two minutes of silence their remembrance and respect for the dead. One friend said that her Israeli boss had told her either to stand up in respect while the siren was heard, or not to come to work at all that day. Another friend said that she went to the workers' restroom at that moment, where she found 12 other Palestinian women. All of them were evading the imposition of honoring the very people who have been persecuting us since the earliest origin of the idea to establish the state of Israel on our homeland.

A second anecdote took place at an Israeli college in Jerusalem, where Palestinian Jerusalemites (Palestinians with Israeli citizenship) and Israeli Jews study. Here, a wallboard was installed as a memorial dedicated to fallen Israeli soldiers so that students could write the name of "their loved ones and light candle in their memory," as the college student union explained. The memorial wall was then found one day with candles extinguished and *Ramadan Kareem* written on the memorial wall board itself. Police and right-wing political parties then became involved in the matter. One Jerusalemite girl was accused of having carried out this "vandalizing" and six others were accused of supporting her; all are currently awaiting punishment. Condemnation of the act is reportedly affecting "all the Arabs" at the college, who are expected to share in general guilt and shame. No one has commented that the presence of the board in the first place erases the memory and the national history of the Palestinians.

Recently, Israel has launched accusations and incitement against Palestinian schools that were brought to the European Union. A written reply to this issue, issued by Federica Mogherini, the High Representative of the European Union for Foreign Affairs and Security Policy, confirmed that a study on Palestinian school curricula is being planned: "Terms of reference for the study are currently being prepared with a view to identifying possible incitement to hatred and violence, and any possible lack of compliance with UNESCO standards of peace and tolerance in education." But no such study is planned for the Israeli curricula! Israelis apparently demand that Palestinian curricula completely erase the map and the history of Palestine and, in its place, teach the history of the European Holocaust to youngsters who are already overwhelmed with the torments of their immediate life experiences.

I am all for academic study and reform of Palestinian curricula—a study examining the extent to which Palestinian curricula teach critical thinking, autonomy and agency and a reform that helps Palestinian youngsters understand their current experience within the full context of genuine Palestinian history. This reform will not resemble the deformed and amputated version of

Palestinian history tailored to donors' "will and values." What is needed is study and reform of our curricula done by Palestinians and for Palestinians.

Recently, the Palestinian Ministry of Education and Higher Education, in the presence of top Palestinian officials such as Mr Azzam and Mr Saeb Erekat, launched a book titled *Our Role Model is Our President*. It features a picture of Mahmoud Abbas on its cover and is said to contain examples of his remarks. These officials first glorified the book and announced that it would be distributed throughout the schools in Palestine. But the initiative received so much criticism and mockery in the scholarly and popular media that the government backed off this project, and announced that the book will not be part of the curricula after all.

This is an agonising time of year for us—when we remember the tragic events that led to the occupation of Palestine and anticipate what is yet to come in the "Deal of the Century." We search within the untold history of the defeated and learn there of the evil of the Zionist project and the international powers who equipped the colonizing Jews in their conquest of the Palestinian nation, the betrayal of the official Arab leadership who disempowered the Palestinians, and the naivete and inadequacy of the Palestinian leadership who placed their trust in this Arab leadership and the Western powers. The Nakba had been initiated many years before the actual establishment of Israel and continues to this very day—reflected in our deep apprehensions regarding the "Deal of the Century" and our realization that power dynamics globally have not fundamentally evolved since these beginnings. The Nakba affects not only Palestinians but the whole Arab world, because the entire region is weakened and undermined by the Israeli occupation, even if the Palestinians just happen to be in the way and must to be killed or transferred to make room for the newest colony of the Western Empires.

The state of Israel was established with ethnic cleansing, massacres and crimes quite similar to those that are nowadays committed by the Islamic State in its path to create yet another religious state. The difference is that Israel has managed to erase memory. Who remembers the Hagana forcing Palestinians to dig their own mass graves in Tantoura, then shooting and burying them there on 22 and 23 May 1948? This is the history of the "most moral army" in the world. The chief terrorists of the past became statesmen and won Nobel prizes—although the wanted poster for Menachem Begin might act as a reminder.

Today, the Eurovision song contest held in Tel Aviv on the anniversary of Israel's crimes of "independence" is an example of the brainwashing strategy that Israel has always used to induce people to forget history—even very recent history, in which the Israeli Army killed 60 and injured 2700 Palestinians in one day when they demonstrated at the border of Gaza at the March of Return in protest of the relocation of the US embassy to Jerusalem.

At a time when the culture and politics of Israel are hypermnestic and super sensitive to its own history, Israel is relentless in its ongoing attack on ours. The war on our history is part of the war on our minds and a muted continuation of ethnic cleansing of the Palestinian nation. We hold memories charged with pain as we hope for the future; it is said that those who don't remember their past are condemned to repeat it.

A Betrayed Generation in Palestine Reveals Post-Oslo Nihilism and Cynicism

Originally published on *Middle East Monitor*, 1 October 2018

More than 55% of Palestinians living in the occupied territories were born after the signing of the Oslo Accords 25 years ago. What is life like for this generation, now that their hopeful dreams of independence and prosperity have been reduced to a nightmare by the ongoing occupation of Palestinian land and the destruction of our social fabric by rival political factions?

Young people in Palestine face a double vulnerability: the universal vulnerability of the adolescent developmental phase as it transitions rapidly from dependence to responsibility, leading to the formation of an individual identity shaped by each individual's particular cognitive and emotional liabilities; and the vulnerability arising from the context of occupation, which limits possibilities and opportunities, jeopardizes personal independence, fragments identity and overwhelms cognitive and emotional resources.

No Palestinian can celebrate Oslo after all that Israel has done to turn its back on its commitments. Washington, the alleged peacebroker, has taken a flagrantly damaging stand against Palestinians through moving the US embassy from Tel Aviv to Jerusalem, closing the PLO's office in the US capital (the only genuine achievement of Oslo), and cutting funds for UNRWA, Palestinian hospitals in occupied East Jerusalem, and other humanitarian programmes.

Oslo prepared our youth for an illusion that ended in shocking disillusion; an even greater disparity between Israelis and Palestinians and an increased dependency of the latter on the former. These outcomes have brought confusion to the hopes, values and sense of meaning which had been shared by the Palestinian people. These failures have brought ambivalence to relationships between them. The result is that many young Palestinians have fallen into nihilism or cynicism.

The statistics demonstrate this. In 2013, the Association for Civil Rights in Israel (ACRI) published a report indicating that the dropout rate for Palestinian students in Israeli-administered schools in Jerusalem was 13% for students for all ages and 36% for 12th grade pupils, whereas the total dropout rate for students in Jewish–Israeli schools in East Jerusalem was only 1%.

A recent study conducted by the Palestinian National Institute for Public Health estimated the prevalence of drug use in Palestine to be 1.8% among males aged 15 and above. Available data indicates that drug use starts at the average age of 17, with an 80% majority of drug users falling between the ages of 18 to 28 years. Media reports, meanwhile, demonstrate how the Israeli police turn a blind eye to drug trafficking, especially in East Jerusalem, where the prevalence at least doubles that in the West Bank; and how drug dealers are protected by the Israeli system through their distance from the Jewish community.

The use of drugs in Palestine brings to mind the 19th century Opium Wars between the British Empire and China, as well as the more contemporary allegations that the CIA participated in cocaine trafficking in Nicaragua, and the FBI was involved in flooding black communities in the US with cheap drugs that resulted in the narcotizing of the youth of these communities and the discrediting of their hopes for social revolution.

General Prosecutor reports show an increase in suicide attempts in Palestine, especially among young people. Over the first nine months of 2017, the police reported 237 cases of suicide attempts in the West Bank, a figure which we know is the tip of the iceberg. Suicide is also on the rise in Gaza. In a study published by the *International Journal of Paediatric and Adolescent Medicine* last year, Taha Itani and colleagues found that the prevalence of suicidal ideation was 25.6% among Palestinian middle-school pupils. This rate is higher than the rates in similar schools internationally, based on surveys of participating countries, which ranged from 15.6 to 23%.

In addition to the important role of individual factors in school dropout, drug abuse and suicidality, there are powerful social and political determinants that promote nihilistic thinking and readily serve as the "straw that broke the camel's back" in overcoming individual resilience to personal problems.

In Palestine, there is a pervasive and commonplace experience of traumatic death, loss and serious injury brought about by political violence. In addition, with very high rates of unemployment and poverty, dim future prospects are likely to contribute to further fears and worries among Palestinian youth. This frame of mind promotes an attitude towards death which focuses on its inevitability, leading to risk-taking and neglect of constructive planning. Clearly, when a person feels worthless in the eyes of the state and of society, she or he loses hope easily and falls back upon regressive withdrawal such as addiction and passivity.

The existential crisis and moral emptiness experienced in Palestine through the mirage of Oslo plays an important role in the loss of healthy desires and motivations toward life itself. At one time, Palestinian society was fortified by faith in its collective cause. Palestinians felt a greater degree of national unity and a sense of confidence in the ability to identify friend from foe. Oslo has undermined these meanings; it is no surprise that young people, especially, suffer from the disintegration of our national ideals and coherent vision of the future.

The youth in Palestine today are being misled in their right to resistance by their own statesmen and by deceptive joint "peace" projects. They are deprived of opportunities for significant social and political engagement. The Youth Development Index of 2016 ranks Palestine among 183 countries at 175 in "Civic Participation" and 148 in "Political Participation". It is no surprise that one finds the youth of Palestine—this most betrayed of generations—at the front lines of the struggle offering endless painful sacrifices. Youth in Palestine compose the majority of those killed, injured, maimed by amputation and injury, and arrested in our violent political context.

Meanwhile, in official Palestinian political bodies, no one is younger than the age of retirement. We have failed to engage our youth, although their participation is crucial to the healthy functioning of state institutions and political parties. This situation is not only pervasive in jokes on social media but also apparent in polls. A recent study conducted by FAFO Foundation as part of the EU-funded Power2Youth initiative, revealed that Palestinians aged 18—29 had low levels of trust in their institutions: only 30% expressed confidence in state security forces, 35% in the police, and 39% in the courts. According to the Global Observatory, only 27% of Palestinian youth expressed confidence in the central government, 12% in the parliament, and—a particular low point—only 8% in political parties. This massive mistrust of social, political and legal institutions can explain why phenomenal "lone wolf" action has become the commonplace modality of resistance in the West Bank.

We are now about to observe World Mental Health day for 2018, an event that chose to highlight the topic of "Young People and Mental Health in a Changing World." This has prompted me to remind the world of the political determinants of mental health in Palestine, particularly for our young people. In addition to the individual medical and therapeutic interventions that must be taken to improve the health of certain individuals among our youth, attention must be given to the larger societal picture. We must develop the necessary policies to create social solidarity, to reduce unemployment and poverty, and to bring quality and meaning to the lives of young people in Palestine. Only then can we provide our youth with opportunities to take on responsibilities constructively, to engage them with hope and to safeguard them from harm.

The Innocence of Those Who Fear
and the Guilt of Those Who Hate

Originally published on *Middle East Monitor*, 14 November 2017

In our stressful state of occupation, there is, among other ills, an essentialist view of Israeli and Palestinian characteristics. In the many public talks that I have given to Westerners about the violation of the rights of Palestinians, one question almost invariably comes up: "What about the fears of the Israelis?" Similarly, how many times have we heard Western media and even the President of the United States speak of "Palestinian hatred"? These words take for granted the guilt of those who "hate" and the innocence of those who "fear." However, the reality is that we cannot understand concerns regarding the fears of the Israelis without dissecting the accusations of "Palestinian hatred."

One problem in this dichotomy is its assumption of a fixed, static state, as if the fears of the Israelis and the hatred of the Palestinians are inborn, permanent traits with no variation among group members. The presumption of eternal and unanimous characteristics serves to maintain the oppressive relationship between the occupier and the occupied and to obstruct political change. To find a way out, the essentialism must be contextualized and deconstructed.

Let us begin by clarifying the disproportionality of the fears of the Israelis with regard to the realistic harm that Palestinians have brought upon them. Israel has long had one of the most powerful armies in the world; it gives "lessons in security" to other nations and exports arms to them for the purpose of oppressing others. Moreover, in order to foster its violent occupation and suppress the natural reflexive resistance on the part of the natives of Palestine, Israel has caged unarmed Palestinians behind walls and appointed colluding Palestinians to maintain order and silence within these cages. By means of long-term and sophisticated strategies to damage Palestinian collective identity, Israel has infiltrated every Palestinian neighbourhood with spies and collaborators. In every previous confrontation, the number of Palestinian casualties has been 100 times the number of Israeli casualties. Thousands of Palestinians are in Israeli prisons, not the other way around; thousands of Palestinian, *not* Israeli, homes have been demolished by Israeli bulldozers; and yet it is the unarmed and stateless Palestinians who are asked to be considerate of Israeli fears.

In view of these facts, it is unjust and insulting when the question of "Israeli fears" is addressed to a Palestinian, insofar as the question itself reveals deep denial of the longstanding history of Israeli violence. The plea for empathy and understanding, when addressed to the victims of Israeli occupation, is absurd, yet the expectation is that Palestinians must demonstrate understanding and offer reassurance for their oppressors' fears. The failure to do so is taken as further evidence of "Palestinian hatred" and confirmation that the Israelis are right to fear them.

I understand very well the traumatic fears caused by the history of the Jews in Europe during the 20th and previous centuries, but why should I, a Palestinian, be called upon to soothe these past fears when I am busy with the traumatic present of occupied Palestine? How can I experience deep empathy for this historical European tragedy when the Israeli threats to my existence and security continue to upstage past events in demanding my urgent attention?

Furthermore, the fear of the Israelis is not simply innocent traumatic heritage; it is a suspect political instrument; a wicked manipulation justifying their cruel treatment of the Palestinians. The invocation of Israeli fears silences protest against the occupation, insisting that all Israelis are implicated in the occupation regardless of their individual hesitations about it. And more evil yet is the fact that this manipulated fear cannot be soothed until the Palestinians disappear completely.

The pretence of fear provides an excuse for crime and absolves "frightened" criminals of responsibility; it falsely attributes the responsibility to the "frightening" victims of the crime instead. Is this not what is implied by the misnomer "Islamophobia"? Why is prejudice and crime directed at Jews called anti-Semitism when prejudice and crime against Muslims—many of whom are also Semites—is not called anti-Muslim hate and a crime? It is called instead the minimizing term "Islamophobia", implying that the hate, racism and criminality of the perpetrator is justified because he or she suffers from anxiety and irrational fears about Islam.

To be fair, a degree of fear on the part of Israelis is appropriate; it's the fear that a tiny proportion of their violence might come back to haunt them, rarely as rockets or a bombing, more often as a Palestinian youth may attempt to punish the Israelis by throwing a stone or pursuing an Israeli soldier with a screwdriver. These things may happen as long as the United Nations and the Palestinian leadership fail to hold the Israelis to account for their crimes.

Attributing fear to the Israelis recruits empathic identification with them, whereas attributing the degrading trait of hatred to the Palestinians provokes repulsion and aversion to them. While there is hatred for the state of Israel among Palestinians, this does not go beyond the adaptive and inevitable hatred that any oppressed and colonized group holds for the collective group that has perpetrated endless crimes against them. Palestinians do not hate Israelis as Jews but as participants in the system responsible for their political oppression. Palestinians are not born with hate in their hearts; hate develops as an appropriate reaction to the totality of the heinous experiences of life under occupation. The people of Palestine are not known for their anti-Semitism; they have welcomed pilgrims from Africa and refugees from Armenia. Many Muslim and Christian Palestinians were married to Jews living in Palestine before the occupation. Like any nation, though, the people of Palestine hate the theft of their land, the pain and the humiliation that the occupation has inflicted upon them. This is, surely, legitimate hate, serving the function of distinguishing harm from safety and motivating resistance to oppression rather than submission to despair.

To expect Palestinians to be free of hate or other negative feelings towards Israel is like expecting a raped woman to have empathy towards her rapist. This would be an example of Stockholm syndrome—a dissociation at best—and more psychologically dangerous than hate itself. This syndrome will eventually result in an internalization of that hate which would then express itself destructively within the oppressed community.

What Israel actually fears is its own dark "Shadow," its enormous but disowned and projected violence and hatred for the Palestinians.

It was not fear, but hatred that permitted Israel to commit massacres which evacuated Palestinian villages and towns by force, and which motivates soldiers to kill handcuffed prisoners and unconscious, wounded Palestinians. It is hatred that incites Jewish settlers to burn Palestinians alive and uproot the ancient olive trees of Palestine. Hate speech is articulated by Israeli soldiers who call Palestinians "beasts on two legs", "drugged cockroaches" and "crocodiles who want more meat." This is hate speech which not only encourages hateful acts committed in the name of the occupation but also legitimizes ethnic cleansing. Isn't that what we must do with cockroaches; get rid of them?

Instead of blaming the Palestinians for their hatred and excusing the Israelis for their fear, a constructive move forward would be to help Israel to distinguish reality from fantasy. This would mean admitting Israeli's own hatred, as well as its greed, and acknowledging that ending the heinous occupation is the only remedy for its fears.

How to Hold Israel Accountable for Torturing Palestinians

Originally published on *Middle East Eye*, 27 March 2024

Torture remains a pervasive reality in Palestine, where countless individuals have endured unspeakable physical and psychological trauma at the hands of Israeli forces. Addressing this grave human rights violation demands a comprehensive approach, including the development of specialized skills for healthcare professionals tasked with documenting and treating survivors. Trained in the Istanbul Protocol for Torture Documentation, I have dedicated myself to equipping fellow professionals with the necessary tools to navigate this challenging terrain. As violence continues to escalate—and as the phenomenon of torture is not restricted to detention centers but witnessed in the streets of the occupied Palestinian territories and filmed on cameras—it is more imperative than ever that we bolster health workers' capacity to document torture experiences professionally, thereby amplifying the voices of survivors in their pursuit of justice.

Context

Since 1967, the Palestinian population has borne the brunt of systematic oppression, with approximately 800,000 individuals subjected to arbitrary detention. Within the confines of Israeli detention centers, Palestinians have routinely faced brutal physical and psychological abuse that meets the stringent criteria for torture set forth by the United Nations. Key elements in torture are the intentional infliction of severe mental or physical suffering by a public official, who is directly or indirectly involved, to achieve a specific purpose. The recent surge in torture incidents, particularly since October 7, serves as a stark reminder of the urgent need to document these atrocities and hold perpetrators accountable before the eyes of the international community.

The experience of torture

The torture tactics employed against Palestinians are as varied as they are barbaric, ranging from crude physical beatings to sophisticated "no-touch" techniques imported from global interrogation practices. Israeli interrogators have also exported to the world specific torture techniques such as "the Palestinian chair." In addition to inflicting excruciating pain through methods such as suspension and simulated drowning, Israeli forces employ psychological warfare, exploiting cultural sensitivities and individual vulnerabilities to amplify the suffering of their victims. Sleep deprivation is an essential part of psychological torture. Reports of sexual abuse, including rape, sodomy and forced nudity, further underscore the depths of depravity to which detainees are subjected. The insidious combination of physical and psychological torture serves not only to punish but also to extract coerced confessions and intelligence, leaving enduring scars on the bodies and minds of survivors, traumatizing their friends and family members, intimidating the whole Palestinian community.

The psychological impact

Central to the efficacy of torture is its capacity to shatter the psychological resilience of its victims, reducing them to a state of utter helplessness and dependency. Through a process of systematic degradation and manipulation, interrogators engineer a reality in which the victim's sense of self is eroded and replaced by a pathological identification with the abuser. This insidious dynamic not only distorts the victims' perception of reality but also undermines their ability to articulate their ordeal coherently. Long after the physical wounds have healed, survivors grapple with a myriad of psychological sequelae, including traumatic stress disorder, depression, and a profound distrust of others. These enduring psychological scars pose serious challenges to the documentation process, as survivors navigate an inner labyrinth of trauma-induced memory deficits, confusion and emotional distress.

Challenges to documentation
The act of documenting torture experiences is fraught with challenges—chief of them being the enduring effects of trauma on survivors' ability to recall and recount their experiences. Memory deficits, coupled with pervasive fear and distrust, often impede survivors' willingness to engage in the documentation process. Moreover, the very act of revisiting traumatic memories can trigger intense emotional distress or avoidance, further complicating efforts to elicit coherent narratives. As healthcare professionals, we must remain attuned to these challenges, employing trauma-informed approaches that prioritize survivors' autonomy and well-being while seeking to uphold their right to truth and justice.

Conclusion
In the face of such abhorrent human rights violations, adherence to the Istanbul Protocol offers a tool of professional resistance, providing a standardized framework for documenting torture

that is grounded in principles of compassion and human dignity. By equipping healthcare professionals with necessary skills and resources, we can empower torture survivors to reclaim agency over their narratives, amplifying their voices in the pursuit of accountability and redress. As we strive to combat torture and uphold the rights of the victims, let us stand in solidarity with survivors, bearing witness to their pain and advocating tirelessly for a future free from oppression and impunity.

Case Report: Imprisonment and torture–triggered psychopathology

Originally published on *Academia.edu*, 2008

Since the beginning of the Israeli occupation of the Palestinian territories in 1967, over 650,000 Palestinians have been detained by Israel. This forms about 20% of the Palestinian population in the Occupied Territories and approximately 40% of the male population since the majority of detainees are men. In my practice in the Community Mental Health sector in the West Bank, I have observed that quite a few of our patients had their first episode of mental illness while they were in detention or just as they were released.

The following is a case report of a 46-year-old man who developed psychosis during his fifth detention. I will first report the story of this patient in particular, and then illuminate this case by taking a broader look at the effects of torture in general.

Family, personal history and premorbid personality

The patient, Jamal, is the third among three brothers and eight sisters. His older brother was killed. His father is deceased. Jamal lives with his mother, his 37-year-old wife and children: two boys and six girls between 18 and 25 years. There is no family history of mental illness. The patient has a high school education. He married at the age of 19, has worked as a laborer, but is currently jobless. Jamal is reported to have been a stubborn, reserved, perfectionist, idealistic man in the past.

Initial mental examination

The patient comes alone to the interview.

He seems very organized, has bits of paper with the names and doses of drugs he uses. He appears very reserved, anxious and has a very polite attitude. Jamal affirms that he is doing "well"—his only problem is unemployment and poor concentration. He denies hallucinations since he's been out of prison. However he believes that some "collaborators" are following him, and that they might be getting information about him from his family. This he "knows" from the clicks he hears sometimes over the phone, and the gestures of neighbours when they come to visit. He seemed very distressed while talking about this, and complains about his wife's and children's "naive" willingness to talk to strangers. The patient is alert, oriented to time, place and person, and has adequate concentration and memory.

In the following sessions, his story unfolds as he talks more about his prison experiences. As he talks about this, he is often in tears. Sometimes, his wife also comes along and gives her side of the story.

History of the disease

Jamal is a former political prisoner. He was held without charge or trial five times. The first was at the age of 14 in 1975 after the death of his older brother who was not even an activist and was killed "by chance" when on his way from school he passed a demonstration. "My brother was wounded by the soldiers and I was arrested. In prison I learnt that my brother had deceased. I remained six months in prison. At the beginning, I was very sad and it was very difficult. When I left I felt that I had grown much older. In 1981, I was in jail again—I still do not know the reason why. That time

I remained six months under interrogation. In the prison I made the decision to get married as soon as I got out—I wanted an ordinary life. I married a few months after I was released. In a year I had the first child. In 1987, I was arrested once more; my wife was pregnant and gave birth while I was in detention. In 1990, I had rather heavy financial expenses and debts and my fourth detention put my family in a serious predicament. All four detentions lasted six months, in each I lived under interrogation and physical and psychological torture."

According to Jamal's wife, he was "normal" as he left prison in the past, though he never used to speak of his experiences there. But in 2003 he was held again, this time for 11 months, and when he returned he had changed. His wife says: "When he came out of prison I was told he became 'crazy' during the last three months of detention. At the beginning I did not believe that, but now I worry much for him. He is very sceptical, he doubts everyone; myself, the children, the neighbours, everyone. He interprets things wrong—if a neighbour visits us, he thinks that he is a spy. He refuses to eat what people bring us. He broke the cell phones, and the satellites, because he thinks we'd better protect ourselves from informers." His wife also thinks that he hears voices. She never sees him speaking alone but she often sees him very concentrated and quiet, as if listening to something or someone. "He sleeps little, and when he sleeps he shouts and speaks about torture. He does not sleep with me anymore, he is impotent. He also eats very little and prepares his food by himself. I really worry about him. He is always tired, often sad, remains all the day in pyjamas. He does not work any more." The fifth detention seemed to have brought about a major shift in Jamal's life. What went wrong this time?

In all detentions he underwent torture, but most severely so the last time. "They tried to force me to confess things that I did not commit. My hands and feet were tied up. I was beaten severely. I was insulted by the filthiest insults related to my religion, wife and mother. There were constant threats to harm my family. My face was covered by a wet bag of draining water. For nights and days I was suspended, sometimes upside down and sometimes on a reversed chair, what they call 'the frog position.' That was extremely painful. I felt as if my limbs were being torn. Then there were the very hot and very cold showers and the imprisonment in a very small room which they call the 'cupboard' or sometimes in another smaller one in the ground which is called the 'coffin.' There was also a third room which was full of collaborators, and which was called 'the room of shame', as some of them commited sexual abuse. Often my stomach hurt out of hunger and I vomited much, in particular when they extended me by the legs and the arms together. Often I had to pee on myself. When I was imprisoned in a total silence and a complete darkness, I lost my sense of time; I could not count the days. Often silence was broken by the cries of people under tortures, yelling of guards or loud Hebrew songs. There I started feeling all my body hurting. The room was very small, I could not move. My joints were all sore. My intestines felt as if torn apart; I felt somehow artificial inside my own body; my viscera were not mine. It was there that I started hearing voices and also seeing the faces of people from outside the prison; I thought they came to the prison to give information about me. I was very frightened and angry. I started shouting at them, I shouted a lot, until the guards attacked my cell and brutalized me because I shouted."

The course of treatment

As Jamal left the prison he had been diagnosed as a case of "schizophrenia." After using typical antipsychotic for six months he reported partial improvement and no hallucinations. However there was no significant change in his mood. Three weeks after his insistence that he was feeling better, he stopped taking the medications. He then started being hostile to his family and neighbours who were "informing about him." Therapeutic doses of antipsychotics and antidepressants were thus started again, in combination with supportive psychotherapy to treat residual symptoms of anxiety, depression, nightmares and constricted affect, and to help Jamal take back his identity and integrate the painful memories.

Torture related psychopathology

The story related above is a case of late-onset affective psychosis, with paranoid delusional ideation and symptoms of major depression. This is a condition we often see in former political prisoners who have been subjected to physical and psychological torture. Kaplan and Sadock (2003) report that "torture is distinct from the other types of trauma because it is inflicted by humans and it is intentional." Kaplan and Sadock's studies revealed a 36% prevalence of PTSD among survivors of torture, as well as high rates of depression and anxiety. Other common psychological complaints included somatization, obsessive compulsive symptoms, hostility, phobia, paranoid ideation and psychotic episodes. Torture has the aim of increasing the suggestibility of the tortured, to impair their judgement and ability to conduct logical arguments against their interrogators, and to confuse what they believe and refute. In his book, *A Question of Torture: CIA Interrogation From the Cold War to the War on Terror*, McCoy discusses a CIA-sponsored research at McGill by Dr Donald Hebb. In this study 22 college students were placed in small, sound-proof cubicles, wearing translucent goggles, thick gloves and a U-shaped pillow around the head. Most subjects quit the study within two days, and all experienced hallucinations and "a deterioration in the capacity to think systematically; subjects were so starved for stimulation that they would even crave interaction with their interrogator", McCoy reports. While institutionalized torture tends to be subtle and easy to conceal, it is designed to violate psychological needs and cause deep damage to psychological structures and breakage of the foundations of normal mental functions. Torture can invade and destroy the subjects' belief in their autonomy as human beings, and destroy their presumptions of interiority, privacy, intimacy. In *Ethics of the unspeakable: Torture survivors in psychoanalytic treatment* Beatrice Patsalides describes how as a result of torture the gap between the "I" and the "me" deepens, and the layer between the "me" and "you" is lost.

Torture includes the deliberate use of extreme stressors, including severe physical pain, inducing psychological pain such as paralyzing fear of pain or death, confusion due to unfulfilled anticipation, violation of deep-seated social or sexual norms, and extended solitary confinement. Techniques like hooding for sensory disorientation, forced nudity, forced standing, cold showers and blindfolding, intimidating detainees with military dogs, withholding food and water, and being pelted with urine or faeces are often reported. Sometimes this degrading treatment is purposefully contradicted with artificial kindness, false favouritism, and grandiose specialness to further mislead the subject and lead to a mutated, disjointed, or discredited personality and belief structure. When the tortured person's physiological needs are controlled by the torturer and only allowed to be expressed in a self-degrading and dehumanizing manner, when emotions of shame, worthlessness, and dependency are induced by a superior, cruel outsider, this can induce psychological regression in the subject by bringing a superior outside force to bear on his or her will to resist.

In his evaluation of victims of torture and other abuses from the Balkan wars, Basoglu showed that psychological torture was as bad as physical torture, and led to similarly high rates of depression and PTSD. What mattered most was the degree to which the victim felt a loss of control. The loss of control over one's life and body brought about by torture is often exacerbated by the disbelief many torture subjects encounter when trying to express what they have been through, especially if they are unable to produce scars or other "objective" proof of their private experience of pain. Torture can also change the mode of relating to reality and the sense of self. Even long after the actual activity is discontinued, some torture victims feel alienated, unable to communicate, relate, attach, or empathize with others. Their basic trust is destroyed and their closest relationships and lifelong support network are disrupted.

As we have seen, a variety of dysfunctions have been attributed to torture, including PTSD, psychosis, depression and anxiety. In my practice, the psychopathology triggered by torture can vary in a wider spectrum, from more subtle symptoms including emotional flatness, social withdrawal, psychotic microepisodes, sexual dysfunction, and recollections of the traumatic events that intrude in the form of nightmares, flashbacks, or distressing associations, to more severe symptoms such as memory disorders, hallucinations, inability to maintain long-term relationships or even mere intimacy, and persistent changes in perception and affect.

I hope my observations can be the precursor for a pilot study to estimate the prevalence of psychopathology among Palestinian former prisoners, compared to that of a non-prisoner population and that of former prisoner populations in other conflict contexts.

About Prisoners

Originally published in French as 'Résistance et resilience' on *Association France Palestine Soidarité*, 9 April 2023

In what context did you meet political prisoners? In prison? On their release from prison? In a professional capacity? At their request?

I meet political prisoners all the time, Since the beginning of the Israeli occupation of the Palestinian territories in 1967, around 800,000 Palestinians have been forcibly detained by Israel. This number comprises about 20% of the entire Palestinian population in the Occupied Territories and about 40% of Palestinian men, since the majority of detainees are male. When in detention, Palestinian prisoners are routinely subject to physical and/or mental mistreatment which meets established UN criteria for torture, although the precise definition and prevalence of torture are subject to politicized debate. Torture clearly presents a major public health threat for Palestinians.

In my clinic, I occasionally see people who come to see me because they suffer from the psychological consequences of torture, a common experience in political detention. More commonly, I see people who come to see me for any psychiatric complaints; they don't even mention that there is political imprisonment in the background; there is an abnormal sense of normalcy regarding this painful experience. The discussion about imprisonment is not put forward spontaneously, it is revealed through the psychiatric intake, as I always ask about traumatic experiences including political imprisonment. I also receive many children, wives who suffer a lot due to the political imprisonment of their family members. I also provided therapy to a boy who was born from a smuggled sperm from prison, he has no identity papers, and he never met with his father, who spends a life sentence in an Israeli prison within 40 km distance from where he lives. I have also been providing psychological support for the beneficiaries, especially women ex-prisoners of Addameer organization, through group and individual sessions. Even when Israel shut down Addameer, together with six other human rights organizations, I continued to provide psychological support online for the beneficiaries. I also have family members and friends who experienced political imprisonment and with whom it is most difficult to talk about this experience, as I don't wear my professional protective shield.

In the Palestinian health care system, is there an offer of individual or collective psychological support, or a possibility of providing psychiatric care to prisoners and their families?

Yes, indeed. We provide more individual support than a collective one. The public health system as well as many community-based NGOs provide free of charge service for individuals, and there are some initiatives to work collectively, but this is more challenging. The stigma associated with mental health problems, as well as the destruction of trust, which is a common experience of a political prisoner, are serious barriers to working in a group setting. Nevertheless, there were several attempts to provide psychological support workshops, stress management skills, and professional development to minor prisoners in a group setting.

In my professional capacity I also use and train other professionals to use a standardized approach to preparing persuasive legal documentation of torture. Developed in 2004, it is commonly called The Instanbul Protocol on the Documentation of Torture.

Each life path is unique. But are there particular profiles that you find in the stories that precede the arrests? In the ways of living through the trials? During administrative detention? During incarceration? Or on release from prison?

People are often detained in the middle of the night with excessive violence of soldiers invading the home, terrifying the whole family and the people in the neighborhood and producing unnecessary damage in properties. There were stories where a father was killed when he interfered as the soldiers were beating the son while arresting him or a mother arrested when she tried to protect her minor. In August 2022, Muhammad AlShahham, 21, was killed at home with a close bullet in the head after soldiers blew the door of his home. Blindfolding the detained is a common practice even with minors, there is no security need for such a practice when a dozen fully armed soldiers escort an unarmed handcuffed adolescent; there is a psychological need, to disorient and control the detainee and break his agency and immediately render him dependent on the soldiers, I guess some soldiers also want to psychologically protect themselves from the gaze of their victim. When transferred to prison, the detainee is often exposed to physical violence, threats and humiliation. During interrogation, psychological torture methods in addition to physical torture are commonly used to break the defenses of the individual. I listened to horrifying details of military interrogation that some of the detainees were exposed to; experiences that are difficult to share in order to not hurt the reader of this interview.

Torture reported by Palestinians commonly involves physical beatings and neglect of basic physical needs. However, reflecting global developments in the techniques of torture (especially input from the United States Central Intelligence Agency), Israeli forces have in addition adopted techniques to inflict pain through so-called "no touch" techniques. These techniques include suspending the victim in mid-air by chaining the hands from above or draping the victim's torso belly-up over a chair seat while chaining the victim's limbs to the chair's four legs. Many frequently utilized techniques of inflicting bodily damage and physical as well as mental suffering are thus disingenuously termed psychological torture, insofar as the torturer does not directly apply the proximate damaging force to the victim; the force of gravity and the victim's own physiology lead to the physical injury and agony arising from so-called "stress positions" and near-death experiences.

Frequently employed psychological techniques include unpredictable periods of isolation in solitary confinement, sensory deprivation through hooding, visual and auditory sensory overload, and sleep deprivation to induce disorientation and cognitive disruption. Specific aspects of Palestinian culture, such as modesty regarding sexuality and a revulsion towards dogs, are exploited in various violations including sexual harrasment and sodomy. Rape is threatened to the detainee's sisters and mothers, as are death threats to family members generally. Nakedness, full body searches, and humiliation of detainees are commonplace. Victims are induced to vomit, and left to soil themselves, to menstruate, and to urinate in the absence of customary standards of privacy and in conflict with personal boundaries and social norms.

A few Palestinian detained were killed during interrogation. I read painful accounts of women like Tahani Abu Dukka and Aysha Aysha AlKurd who were medically neglected and forced to abort their babies during administrative detention in the book *Making*

Women Talk, London 1992. The book also describes the added torture techniques reserved for women prisoners. The whole process of detention interrogation is designed to mentally breakdown the activists and intimidate the Palestinian community and inflict guilt and paranoia. Torture experiences are often repeated daily over a period of months and years and throughout repeated episodes of detention. It is obvious that well-recognized, long-term and sometimes lifetime consequences of torture—psychiatric syndromes including PTSD and other dissociated states, psychotic symptoms, paranoia, depression, anxiety, and deteriorated cognitive, psychological, and social functioning—tend to undermine the capacity to remember and narrate events. The resultant combinations of deficits and psychological defenses interfere with the survivor's memory, his tolerance of reactivating memories of torture through describing it to others, and his hope of court redress. The experience of torture thus typically results in profound damage to those very ego functions upon which conveying a coherent personal narrative history depends: trust in others, optimism regarding the future, accurate recall of events, a sense of personal efficacy, and an orderly integration of past experience. These have been the findings of clinicians and workers involved in the documentation, the treatment and rehabilitation of torture victims in Palestine and globally.

How can you describe and qualify the impact of these arrests and imprisonments on the family? If there are differences, what are the causes?

I encountered some ex-prisoners who are left with pervasive mistrust and isolation following their experience. Some parents of minors in Jerusalem have a total confusion about roles when they have to act as guardians for the home imprisonment of their boys. Some wives were anguished for the detention of their husbands and, after a delay, apprehensive that another man is about to be released from prison. I encountered fathers coming out of prison after many years not finding their old place in the family. There is an immense destructuring of the individual and his family behind the superficial glorification of the experience.

In Palestine the system of mass arrests is also a "collective punishment"; a way for Israel to break down minds, relationships and the social fabric. How does this affect individuals and society? What do you think about the goals of the Israeli governments in carrying out this policy?

In addition to its goals of punishment of individuals and intimidation of the community, imprisonment and torture are routinely coupled with interrogation to obtain a confession and/or information regarding real or alleged plans and the identity of others who are alleged or suspected of involvement. The relationship between the interrogator and the victim is often highly elaborate and constructed especially to undermine the victim's normal, mature psychological functioning through exploiting individual vulnerabilities. The interrogator functions as the sole channel between the victim and reality, reducing the victim to a state of regressive helplessness and total dependency. Holding the victim responsible for his own suffering is a standard aspect of this approach. The combination of delirium and terror regularly and rapidly induces distortions in the victim's reality-testing and his grip on human meaning. These approaches encourage a pathological identification with the interrogator and his goals, a process historically termed brainwashing. The relationship between interrogator and torture victim can be thus intensely personal and may develop the complex character of other abusive intimate relationships characterized by lying, gas-lighting, sadistic seduction, manipulation and perversion.

We can not really dissociate the individual and collective consequences of imprisonments, Israeli military law is designed to give a false impression of the lawfulness of the occupation and to incriminate any Palestinian agency for resistance and defiance. The cost is huge for certain individuals and their families, the younger the prisoner, the more damaging are the effects on the prisoners and the society.

The unusual victories of the few prisoners who earned their freedom through their hunger strike and the outstanding escape of six Palestinian prisoners from Israeli jail in 2021 through a tunnel destroys the illusion of the Israeli omnipotence. It proves that Palestinian detainees continue to enlighten the spark of the liberation movement of the Palestinian people.

About Resistance and Resilience

The Palestinian Resistance:
Its legitimate right and the moral duty

Originally published on *Miftah*, 10 November 2003

The overwhelming and ceaseless atrocities of Israel's government leave most Palestinians with little opportunity to reflect on the moral aspect of our resistance. Most often our reactions to events are immediate, instinctive and emotional. The few who still manage to consider the moral, political and strategic aspects of our struggle may find themselves all but stymied by the contradictions, the lack of choice, and the damage done by war to both reason and conscience.

How can Palestinian resistance be fairly assessed then, with due consideration given to the entire history of the Israeli–Palestinian conflict? The occupation of Palestine is based on a 19th century ideology that denied the very existence of the Palestinian people and pursued a colonial agenda asserting divine claims to a "land without a people." In response to this "theo-colonial" aggression, the Palestinian resistance adopted the strategy of "a protracted people's war" to regain recognition as a dispossessed, rather than "nonexistent" nation.

To this day, Palestinians still have no state or armed forces. Our occupiers subject us to curfews, expulsions, home demolitions, legalized torture, and a highly imaginative assortment of human rights violations. No justifiable comparison can be drawn between the level of official accountability to which Palestinans are held for the actions of a few individuals and the responsibility for the systematic and intense violence against the entire Palestinian population practiced with impunity by the state of Israel. The American media call our search for freedom "terrorism," thus casting the Palestinian in the role of the international prototype for the terrorist. This has shaped Western public consciousness and resulted in an international bias that tends to describe instances of violence against Palestinian civilians in neutral language, reducing Palestinian losses to mere faceless statistics, while using emotional language and visuals to describe Israeli losses.

This distortion of the Palestinian resistance has clouded all reasonable dialogue. Many of our efforts to defy the arbitrary rules of the occupier are reflexively dismissed as "terrorism," and we are always expected to apologize for and condemn Palestinian resistance—despite the lack of agreement on a definition of terrorism, and the fact that the right to self-determination by armed struggle is permissible under the United Nations Charter's Article 51, concerning self-defense.

Why is the word "terrorism" so readily applied to individuals or groups who use homemade bombs, but not to states using nuclear and other internationally prohibited weapons to ensure submission to the oppressor? Israel, the United States and Britain should top the list of terrorism-exporting states for their use of armed attacks against non-combatants in Palestine, Iraq, Sudan and other parts of the world. But "terrorism" is a political term used by the colonizer to discredit those who resist—as the Afrikaaners and Nazis named the Black and French freedom fighters, respectively.

There also is a trend among those who oppose Palestinian resistance to use the term "jihad" as a synonym for terrorism. In doing so, they reduce the meaning of jihad to mere death. Jihad is a rich concept that includes struggling against one's lesser self, the effort to do good deeds, actively opposing injustice, and being patient in times of hardship. It is not about violence against God's creatures, or not fearing death in defending the rights of God's creations. Violence can, however, be a rational human's means of defense. When a woman reacts violently when threatened with rape, that is a form of jihad.

Moreover, jihad is an Islamic value—and not all Palestinian fighters are Muslims. The reason why young, sincere altruistic Palestinians blow themselves up is a secret they take with them to the grave. Perhaps it is the strange fruit of revenge growing in the fertile soil of oppression and occupation, or their profound protest against merciless cruelty; or a desperate attempt at attaining equality with Israelis in death, since it is impossible for them in life. Those who live under inhuman conditions all their lives are, unfortunately, capable of inhuman acts. What is left for the homeless thousands in Rafah except their resistance? It is not Islam; it is human nature, shared by religious, secular and agnostic Palestinian men and women. Certainly, our women bombers do not die in the expectation of 70 virgins awaiting them in Paradise.

Another factor influencing Palestinian resistance is the gloomy history of peace talks and the lack of international support. Negotiations with Israel have given us nothing but promises of autonomy over our impoverishment, while enforcing the will of the powerful and establishing illegalities, as the basis for a lasting settlement. The most glaring absence in this peace process was an honest peace broker. The United Nations has been unable to take steps to ensure the implementation of Palestinian rights. The world has offered not a single remedy for the numerous wounds the Palestinians have suffered; Washington repeatedly has used its veto in the Security Council to thwart the broad consensus calling for an international monitoring presence in the West Bank and Gaza. The relentless denial of Palestinian rights without an effective verbal or actual international response has left us acutely aware that self-defense is our only hope.

International law grants a people fighting an illegal occupation the right to use "all necessary means at their disposal" to end their occupation, and the occupied "are entitled to seek and receive support" (I quote here from several United Nations resolutions). Armed resistance was used in the American Revolution, the Afghan resistance against Russia (which the US supported), the French resistance against the Nazis, and even in the Nazi concentration camps, or, more famously, in the Warsaw Ghetto.

Palestinian resistance arises out of a similarly oppressive situation. The degree of violent response varies from case to case—indeed, in many instances resistance is mainly nonviolent. Despite all the odds against them, people resiliently continue to live, study, pray and plant crops in occupied land. In a few cases, they actively resist and resort to violence. This violent resistance may be defensive (and, thus, to my mind, morally acceptable), such as the resistance of the Jenin refugee camp fighters as Israeli death machines approached; or it may take the form of unacceptable offensive acts, such as the bombing of Israeli civilians celebrating a Passover meal.

In all cases, however, it is individual Palestinians who choose the form of resistance, and the choices they make should not characterize the entire nation. Also, as we have seen, both peaceful and violent resistance are met with sanctioned, deliberate state violence by the democratic and free Israeli government and its forces.

The death of American peace activist Rachel Corrie is evidence enough of that.

"Where is the Palestinian Gandhi?" some people wonder. Our Gandhis are either in prison, in exile or in graves. Nor do we have a population in the hundreds of millions. We are 3.3 million unarmed, defenseless individuals facing six million Israelis, virtually all of them soldiers or reservists. This is not industrial colonization; the Israelis are practicing ethnic cleansing to secure the land for Jews alone.

It is ironic that few of those who exhort Palestinians to emulate Gandhi question Zionism, the root cause of the Israeli occupation. In 1938, however, Gandhi himself questioned the premise of political Zionism. "My sympathy does not blind me to the requirements of justice," he said. "The cry for the national home for the Jews does not much appeal to me. The sanction for it is sought in the Bible and in the tenacity with which the Jews have hankered after their return to Palestine. Why should they not, like other peoples of the earth, make that country their home where they are born and where they earn their livelihood?"

Gandhi clearly rejected the idea of a Jewish state in the Promised Land by pointing out that the "Palestine of the Biblical conception is not a geographical tract."

Violent resistance arises from an inhuman military occupation, one that levies punishment arbitrarily and without trial, denies the possibility of livelihood, and systematically destroys the prospects of a future. The Palestinian people have not gone to another people's homeland to kill or dispossess. Our ambition is not to blow ourselves up in order to terrify others. We are asking for what all other people rightfully have—a decent life in the land of our birth.

What is most troubling about the criticism of our resistance is that it cares little for our suffering, our dispossession, and the violation of our most basic rights. When we are murdered, these critics are unmoved. Our peaceful, everyday struggle to live a decent life makes no impression on them. When some of us succumb to retaliation and revenge, the outrage and condemnation is directed at us all. Israeli security is deemed more important than our right to a basic livelihood; Israeli children are seen as more human than ours; Israeli pain more unacceptable than ours. When we rebel against the inhuman conditions imposed upon us, our critics dismiss us as terrorists, enemies of human life and civilization.

But it is not to appease our critics that we must revisit our resistance. It is because we care about Palestinian morality and morale.

International law and the historical precedent of many nations sanction the right of a people suffering from colonial oppression to take up arms in their freedom struggle. Why should it be different in the case of Palestinians? Is not the point of international law that it is universal? Americans claim life, liberty and the pursuit of happiness as their most fundamental human rights. It is fitting that the right to life should be mentioned first. After all, without the right to remain alive, to be safe from attack, to defend oneself against attack, the other rights become meaningless. Fundamental to that right is exercising the right of self-defense.

We Palestinians continue to face a brutal occupation with exposed chests and empty hands. I believe in dialogue in the Israeli–Palestinian encounter, but negotiations should never be the only option; they must go hand-in-hand with resistance to the occupation. While the Israelis talk to us they continue to build settlements and hastily construct a wall that will further constrict and violate our rights. Why should we abandon our right to resist and remain living in the realm of the murderously absurd?

To live under oppression and submit to injustice is incompatible with psychological health. Resistance not only is a right and a duty, but is a remedy for the oppressed. Even if not as a strategic, pragmatic option, we should resist as an expression of—and insistence on—our human dignity. Violent resistance must always be in defense, and as the last resort. It is important, however, to distinguish between permissible (military) and impermissible (civilian) targets, and to set limits for the use of arms. Nor must the oppressor be exempt from these same principles.

The history of our resistance must be explored and assessed from the perspectives of law, morality, experience and politics, taking timing and context into account and with due regard for human rights, international law and widely shared norms of behavior. Palestinians must be creative in providing effective peaceful alternatives for resistance that can invite the progressives of the world to join our struggle.

Ultimately, the strength of the Palestinian plight lies in its moral, humanitarian characteristics; it is to our benefit to find moral, humanitarian means to protect that strength.

Palestinian Sumud: 'Man shall not live on bread alone'

Originally published on *Middle East Monitor*, 20 July 2015

The Palestinian elections of 2006 displeased Western powers. In the aftermath of the ensuing economic boycott of Palestine, our president told us that "if we have to choose between bread and democracy, we choose bread." However, the baker Khader Adnan thinks and behaves otherwise, exemplifying the principle that "Man shall not live by bread alone." Adnan has endured two long and perilous hunger strikes in Israeli detention since 2013. The first was triggered by torture and humiliating mistreatments; the interrogators made sexual innuendos about his wife, mocked his faith and his physique, ripped out his beard, and put dirt from their shoes on his moustache. Adnan prevailed in both hunger strikes, leading to his liberation from prison and bringing world attention to the plight of Palestinian political prisoners in Israeli administrative detention who are held without charge or trial for six-month periods that can be renewed indefinitely.

Israel did not triumph and Gaza was not broken
Despite the siege and neglect, the Gaza strip remains a center of innovation; recently, gluten-free flour for patients suffering with celiac disease—an ingredient that has not been available in Gaza due to the siege—has been developed and made available there by two researchers at Al Israa University. Young people have constructed machines to assist persons who have been paralyzed as well as designed engines and tools for the detection of land mines. The many years of

closure and the increasing levels of violence brought against the population during the last three wars have failed to break the will of the people there. Today, one year on from the destructive 51-day war that left over 100,000 people homeless, Gaza is still patiently waiting for reconstruction; but waiting in steadfastness.

Jerusalemites: Citizens of nowhere

Living well in Jerusalem is a challenge, since the occupation not only denies us citizenship, assigns us a fragile status as temporary residents, and imposes regulations that threaten our residency, homes and income, but also imposes fines and taxes that have the goal of driving us from our home town. Laws make marriage to a "non-Jerusalemite" a pretext for eventual loss of residency. Nevertheless, during the month of Ramadan and the Eid holiday, when Jerusalem was visited by many Palestinians both from the West Bank and holding Israeli citizenship, we were able to enjoy moments of delight and celebration that emphasizes the Palestinian essence of this hijacked city. Social media were filled with selfies of people who managed to arrive in Jerusalem, some though hidden tunnels and by climbing ladders over the separation wall. People posed with banners carrying the names of friends and family members who had been denied access to the city. These images transcend the trendy superficiality of the typical selfie photo and symbolize our sense of rootedness and belonging. Although Jerusalemites are citizens of nowhere, few of us would trade our home town for anywhere in the world.

On the meaning of Sumud

Such are the experiences associated with the Palestinian concept of "sumud." While it is difficult to come up with an inclusive, all-en-compassing definition of this term, there are countless distinctive examples of it as an individual and collective attitude in extreme situations as well as in everyday life. While terms like "resilience" and "adversity-advanced development" are currently popular in positive psychology, Palestinians have used the term *Sumud* since the time of their defiance of the British mandate. The term has taken on varied meanings at different states of the Palestinian struggle and in response to complex events: massive displacement, life under occupation, life as a Palestinian with Israeli citizenship, imprisonment and exile. While resilience is a concept oriented towards a state of mind, Sumud expresses both a state of mind and an orientation to action.

Sumud then is not just the capacity for survival or the ability to bounce back to cope and adapt to stress and adversity. Sumud is accomplishing these things in addition to maintaining a steadfast defiance to subjugation and occupation. Sumud is not an inborn trait or the consequence of a single life event, but a system of skills and habits that are learned and can be developed. It forms the basis of a lifestyle of endurance; holding onto the land like a deeply rooted olive tree, preserving one's identity, pursuing autonomy and agency, preserving the Palestinian narrative and its culture in the face of elimination.

It is about the self-sufficiency of farmers who subsist on their own limited production while refraining from consuming Israeli prod-ucts; it is reflected in the labor of construction workers who reject the temptation to build Israeli settlements and accept the reduced income available from providing construction for Palestinians; it is seen in the generative capacity of parents whose commitment starts with the birth of a child, but continues by caring for and educating the child to be a decent Palestinian in the face of the threatened annihilation of the Palestinian nation. When the occupation uproots our olive trees, we plant many others; when they demolish our homes, we reconstruct new ones; when they close our schools, we create makeshift schools; when they obscure our history, we engage in witnessing, remembering and documenting. When they fragment us with stratifying colors of identity papers, car plates, and conflicting political parties, we act to build ties of solidarity through collective action that maintains the coherence of the community.

Sumud is not accepting the status quo, tolerating corruption, and enjoying handouts. For many years, in the name of supporting the Sumud of the Palestinians living on occupied land, 5% of the salaries of hundreds of thousands of Palestinian workers in the Gulf was deducted every month by the Aid Fund of the Palestinian Liberation Organisation; some of that money was misused as handouts without development planning and distributed with the purpose of promoting political polarisation. Much of that money was wasted by corruption. When the political winds moved against Palestinians in the Gulf, many lost their jobs and homes. The workers suffered due to the misbehavior of the Palestinian leadership and there was no Sumud money to support them during that predicament.

A government of Sumud: Beyond the antagonism of armed resistance and security coordination

Over the last few months, the Palestinian security forces have arrested hundreds of university students, syndicalists, and journalists from opposition parties—all for "security reasons." While

Khader Adnan prevailed in his hunger strike against the Israeli authorities, Islam Hammad has not yet won his 100-day hunger strike in Palestinian prisons. The Palestinian government creates real obstacles for the people in achieving Sumud and disturbs their capacity to remain focused on the Israeli occupation. While the Oslo accords have created a glass ceiling for Palestinian resistance, there is still some space for the Palestinian government to become a Sumud government, rather than of a government of subcontractors who spare the occupation from facing its responsibilities and do their dirty work at a cheaper price.

All talks about unity government are meaningless without re-conceptualising and reforming the role of the government as genuinely transformative—proceeding according to an inclusive national agenda for liberation without favoritism, nepotism and corruption.

It is the responsibility of the a national unity government to promote the Sumud of the people in the face of occupation, polarisation, corruption and moral degradation. It is the job of the government to enhance the survival of Palestinians on their occupied lands and to preserve the Palestinian identity of the exiled; it must advance the human rights and national objectives of the Palestinian people; it must promote economic survival for all in the face of de-development, consumerism and the growing economic gap between a tiny elite class and an impoverished majority. A Sumud government can preserve our national dignity, in spite of deliberate efforts to bring degradation and humiliation upon Palestinians; it can impact international solidarity with Palestine, because Sumud and solidarity are synergetic values that augment one another's momentum and impact.

The choice of Sumud is not easy or pain-free and does not mean the absence of negative emotions in the face of loss. Rather, Sumud means maintaining optimism, moral and social solidarity while dealing with grim realities and oppressive structures. It is, in effect, like the experience of Khader, Islam and many others; that painful position of searching for our lost freedom with the hope that we will find it one day.

Resistance to Israel's Occupation is an Essential Element in the Recovery of the Occupied Mind

Originally published on *Middle East Monitor*, 18 May 2021

Israel has imposed military occupation, settler-colonialism, and an apartheid regime upon a multitude of fragmented Palestinian communities, thereby creating, sustaining, and contributing to grave health and mental health issues. These are caused directly through inflicting physical and psychological distress, environmental violence and hazards, and targeting medical providers and services; and indirectly through retarding economic growth, disrupting social functioning, and hindering development efforts or improving healthcare provision.

It has been claimed that among all the countries bordering the Eastern Mediterranean, the one with the greatest burden of morbidity due to mental illness is Palestine (Charara et al., 2017). Mental illness in Palestine represents one of its most significant public health challenges, as it occurs in the context of chronic occupation and exposure to violence (WHO, 2019). According to the Humanitarian Needs Overview in 2020, an estimated half-a-million adults and children suffer from mild, moderate, and severe psychosocial distress and mental disorders in occupied Palestine. There is no doubt that Israel's occupation is harmful to the Palestinian mind.

However, this research does not indicate harms measured beyond the level of the individual; that is, the collective harms that affect our relationships within society and with others.

The occupation not only attacks the bodies and brains of those who are affected individually but also attacks the social fabric, the norms, the symbolic representations, and the collective identity of Palestinian society.

Collective consequences of the occupation include internalized oppression, prevalent mistrust throughout the community, and low collective self-confidence and self-esteem. Further consequences are the loss of subjectivity and the presence of self-objectification, the loss of a sense of community agency, an acceptance of inefficacy and status of passive victimhood, as well as an impaired collective functioning and achievement.

Palestinian resistance as expressed in its various forms—from writing slogans on walls to launching rockets—is usually undertaken by individuals acting in the name of the group as a whole. We cannot ignore the impact of this resistance at the collective level, insofar as it has the potential to repair the emotional erosion of the community brought about by oppression. Resistance can move people from conditioned learned helplessness to hopefulness.

Palestinian resistance stems neither from racism nor national chauvinism, nor from political and economic interests, but from deep psychological factors—a need for cognitive coherence instead of dissonance and a need to be active in rejecting oppression through striving for justice and a genuine empathy with those who are oppressed. This resistance represents moral, symbolic, and spiritual values that are crucially important to those who are deprived of material and tangible rights.

Resistance has a humanizing influence, acting against the dynamic of objectification at both the individual and the collective level. It is perceived by Palestinians as a legitimate human right and a moral duty. We may argue about what forms of resistance we should take and at what times it should be enacted, but this argument must be an internal Palestinian debate that cannot be decided for us by others, especially those who have never supported us or defended our rights.

People often ask, "Doesn't the Palestinian resistance backfire and bring more losses to Palestinians?" As I write, Israeli aggression against the Palestinians in Gaza is killing and wounding hundreds of people of all ages, and destroying their homes and infrastructure. As I write, Palestinian rockets cause a much lesser degree of damage in Israel and loss of Israeli lives. As I write, three of my professional colleagues have just been killed along with their children, buried under the rubble in Gaza. As I write, armed Israeli settlers roam around and fire shots in the neighborhood where my family lives.

I understand, though, that the resistance of the oppressed does not subscribe to the usual calculation of risks and benefits that characterize business or economic logic. It cannot be judged merely by its end results. The journey of resistance is dignifying in itself, even in the absence of the achievement of desired goals. It is resistance for a decent life, not death. When Palestinian protesters and Israeli settlers were demonstrating and opposing each other on the streets of Jerusalem recently, the Palestinians chanted "Freedom, liberation," while the Israelis chanted "Death to the Arabs, burn their villages." Above all, the motivation involved in resistance to oppression maintains a positive concept of an imagined future and thus rejuvenated hope for liberation.

Moreover, if Palestinian resistance is the remedy for the collective trauma of the people of Palestine, international solidarity is also rehabilitative and therapeutic for both Palestinians and those who support them. Solidarity validates the humanity of Palestinians and acknowledges their feelings and subjectivity; it nourishes their aspiration to be agents and actors for change. It also has the potential to generate mutual and global activism for justice.

It is a shame that some supposedly democratic governments, such as that in France, are preventing demonstrations from taking place in solidarity with Palestine, arresting the organizers and imposing fines on participants. Despite this, the current Palestinian resistance is the well-spring of struggle against oppressive powers. It shall flourish within and beyond occupied Palestine.

From Palestine To The US We Must Defend People's Right To Breathe

Originally published on *The Palestinian Information Center*, 17 June 2020

We have emerged from the global solidarity brought about by the Covid-19 crisis to return to our familiar state of disunity in the struggle against oppressive power domination and fascist politics.

In *Black Skin White Masks* Frantz Fanon explains the revolt in Indochina: "It is not because the Indo-Chinese has discovered a culture of his own that he is in revolt. It is because 'quite simply' it was in more than one way becoming impossible for him to breathe."

In her 2017 film *Beyond the Frontlines* French director Alexandra Dols also uses the metaphor of breathlessness to convey the Palestinian experience under occupation. In the film's opening she features me in conversation with an Israeli psychoanalyst who challenges me to empathize with Israeli needs. I reply: "We live in a reality where the more Israelis breathe, the more Palestinians choke."

Throughout the film we hear Palestinians gasping for air: during interrogation in prisons at the Qalandiya checkpoint and under bombardment in Gaza.

It is no wonder that George Floyd's cries of "I can't breathe" have provoked so much reaction in Palestine. He uttered these words while being suffocated under the knee of a police officer and amid the approving gaze of fellow officers, a technique commonly used against Palestinians.

Indeed, Israel has developed a flourishing industry of training international police in the utilization of such fatal techniques. Palestinians' sympathetic identification with Floyd's breathlessness is not only due to the effortless choking of a Black man by a white police officer; it also resonates with the Israeli "no-touch technique" in which people are suspended in positions where the weight of their own bodies inflict pain and damage possibly causing them to die alone.

Institutional racism

In both the US and Palestine such acts are not restricted to an individual police officer who is quick on the trigger or to a particular victim. They are pervasive outcomes of group dynamics and institutional racism that permits a sustained pattern of killing on the basis of ethnicity colour or group membership.

Examples include the recent killing in Jerusalem of Iyad al-Halak, a Palestinian man diagnosed with autism. He was shot and left on the ground to bleed to death in spite of his caregiver's efforts to explain to Israeli police that he had a disability—and despite his cries of "I'm with her."

About two weeks prior, psychiatric patient Mustafa Younis was killed at the hospital where he was seeking treatment. After a violent confrontation with security guards Younis was disarmed and lying on the ground; he was then shot with several bullets in front of his mother.

We can learn two things from these recent killings. Firstly, like the casual killing of Floyd racially motivated killings of Palestinians are commonplace—even as Israel brags about normalizing relations with Arab countries.

Israel acts according to the motto that a "good Arab is a dead Arab." Many Palestinians have been shot in the back or upper body with a story fabricated to legitimize the killing. There have been allegations of planted knives and other evidence to implicate Palestinian youth and of camera footage hidden when it contradicts the official narrative.

Secondly, a violent political context not only generates psychiatric patients but also creates easier victims out of them. I know people who had psychiatric issues and were killed because their paranoid delusions made them carry a knife or their limited cognitive abilities made them underestimate realistic risks, or their irritability made them fight back when beaten or humiliated by soldiers.

The reaction to the terrifying killings of people such as Floyd, Younis and Halak must not be restricted to demanding justice for the victims and their families. Their deaths should fuel a wider struggle against racism and against police and political violence.

Our response must embrace a wider solidarity to defend the right to breathe—for all humankind.

Palestine: Therapy as an act of national liberation

Originally published on *Atlas of Wars*, 17 July 2023

Seventy-five years have passed since the violent events of 1948, when two thirds of the Palestinian population were driven from their land and homes by Israeli forces. Since then, the violence has not stopped but has increased on several occasions: a few months ago there were more attacks, including those in Turmus Aya and in Jenin. The strikes on the Jenin refugee camp, an occupied town in the north of the West Bank, claimed the lives of 12 of the 11,000 refugees living there and reopened a major wound in a town that was the scene of one of the worst clashes of the second intifada, or Palestinian uprising, of the 2000s.

Operation Home and Garden by the Israel Defence Forces (IDF) is the largest in 20 years. UN Secretary-General António Guterres has condemned Israel's 'excessive use of force' in the operation which left more than 100 civilians injured, forced thousands to flee, damaged schools and hospitals, and cut water and electricity supplies. He criticized Israel for preventing medical care and aid workers from reaching those in need, and reminded Israel that 'as an occupying power, it has a responsibility to ensure that civilians are protected from all acts of violence.' Meanwhile, internal protests continue in Israel against the judicial reform, which limits the power of the Supreme Court to rule against the legislature and executive. A moment of national pause, but one that does not lessen the military pressure in the West Bank and Gaza.

More than half of the Palestinian population shows symptoms

of depression, according to a recent World Bank study. Dr Samah Jabr, psychiatrist, psychotherapist and head of the Mental Health Department at the Palestinian Ministry of Health, explains how the trauma inflicted on the population has always been on the political agenda of the occupying power, and warns against the data in the report, highlighting the political significance of pathologizing the occupied as a further strategy of elimination.

Dr Jabr, a World Bank study on Palestinian mental health was recently published. It paints an alarming picture, with 50% of the West Bank population suffering from depression, and as much as 70% in Gaza. What do you think?

Like other colonisers and occupiers in the world, Israelis treat the colonized as either barbaric and savage or sick and inferior. One way of making them inferior is to portray them as psychologically inadequate, to pathologize them. That is why we have to be wary of all these reports that pathologize the Palestinian experience and portray Palestinians as having psychological disorders rather than pointing to the real cause of psychological suffering. The study done by the World Bank and the Palestinian Bureau of Statistics says that Palestinians have depression, but in fact Palestinians have immense levels of psychological suffering. The problem with this study is that it does not distinguish between emotional distress and mental disorder on the one hand, and depression as a mental health problem on the other. They used the World Health Organization's WHO-5 questionnaire, which indicates that people who score positive on the questionnaire need further assessment. It doesn't identify people with depression. There is a problem with the interpretation of this survey. A more serious study in 2019 suggests that in countries suffering from political violence, the prevalence of mental health disorders is 22.1%.

How can we describe the situation?

The Western world knows very little about what is happening here, but you probably remember how Daesh, the militancy of the Islamic State, dispossessed and expelled certain minorities from their villages. This is how Palestine was evacuated, in acts similar to what happened when the militants of the Islamic State evicted people from villages in Iraq. This is how towns were expelled in Palestine in 1948, and until today we see Israeli gangsters attacking and terrifying people, so that the traumatic history of Palestine is repeated and there is continuity. That is why I argue that we do not have PTSD in Palestine. We have an ongoing, repetitive, historical, collective trauma that is passed on from one generation to the next, and the Israelis make sure that they traumatize every generation. Most of the victims in Jenin were very young. They were born after the great traumatic event of 2002. The oldest are 21, maybe 23. So they make sure that every generation is exposed to at least one major traumatic event.

How can therapy help people?

Man-made trauma aims to make us helpless and hopeless, and we try to generate hope and maintain our ability to act despite all the difficulties. This is how we survive. We also know that taking care of people psychologically, supporting them and freeing them from the feeling of helplessness and hopelessness caused by traumatic events is also a contribution to the national liberation struggle.

President Abu Mazen has asked the UN and the international community to intervene urgently to force Israel to stop the evacuation in Jenin. What is the expected reaction?

The Palestinians have always experienced that the international community is unable or uninterested in protecting them, including the Palestinian leadership. The inability of the United Nations and the Palestinian leadership to protect the Palestinians creates a void that can be filled by the actions of some young people who are so angry about what is happening. They take on the responsibility to act on behalf of the group and try to do something to liberate Palestine, to force Israel to pay a price for its actions.

What do you think of the protests in Israel against judicial reform? Do these internal disturbances take pressure off the offensive against the Palestinians?

Every time there is a lack of consensus, they attack the Palestinians in order to create more cohesion within the Israeli community.

As for the protests, I think an occupation that looks like a democracy is worse for the Palestinians than an occupation that looks like an autocracy. It annoys me that the international community is more interested in Israel's internal politics than in what Israel is doing for the Palestinians. It ignores reporting important news about Palestine and how Palestinians are treated by the occupation and shows more interest and focus on the details of Israeli domestic politics.

Have mental health professionals around the world supported you so far?

As I developed my career as a mental health professional, I wanted to believe that mental health professionals would be more sensitive to justice, equality and liberation. This is true, except in Palestine. Mental health institutions were vocal about Ukraine, but when we talked about Palestine they were silent. Every time we talked about Palestine, they reminded us of the principles of neutrality and impartiality. They completely forgot about them when it came to Ukraine. I was at the Global Mental Health Summit, where Olena Zelenska was given the space to open the summit and to talk about her country.

There is this underlying support. Palestinians have a different tan and colour, a different physiology to the global north and they are Muslims and there is also racism and islamophobia which makes support for Palestine less likely. But there are good-hearted people and we have set up networks with international organisations, including the UK–Palestine Mental Health Network and the US–Palestine Mental Health Network, and we are setting up another network in Italy. These are networks of mental health professionals, representing individual mental health professionals, who are trying to educate themselves and others around them about the Palestinian situation and the impact of the occupation on the mental health of Palestinians, and they are trying to challenge the occupiers from a mental health point of view.

The Palestinian Cause in Jihadist Ideology: Between fact and fiction

Originally published on *Middle East Monitor*, 9 July 2019

A commitment to Palestine binds together many Arab, Muslim and other marginalized minorities in the West, generating strong emotional, ideological and political support. The nature of this bond often goes beyond issues of kinship or religious connection to involve a common underlying experience of political alienation.

Radical jihadist groups, however, have exploited the Palestinian cause for their own ends. In this contradictory context, the French government has taken measures recently to penalize the expression of non-violent criticism of Zionism and to persecute activists supporting the Boycott, Divestment and Sanctions (BDS) movement; these measures impair the exercise of fundamental human rights and contribute to extremist "radicalisation." I would argue that freedom of expression regarding the Israeli occupation of Palestine can contribute to resilience-building among marginalized communities in France, while also thwarting anti-Semitism and other manifestations of "radicalization."

It is beyond the scope of this article to review all of the literature relevant to this topic, such as the biographies of the Salafi jihadist leaders; or to trace how the issue of Palestine affected the historical trajectory of transnational jihadism. The opinions expressed here are nevertheless informed by the few research materials available on the matter and by the most important statements and videos referring to Palestine that have been produced by the leadership of Al-Qaeda and Daesh (ISIS).

I cannot claim absolute objectivity, as I am not indifferent about Palestine and Islam. Indeed, researching this topic has been especially distressing for me because of the great similarities that I find between the traumatizing propaganda and conduct of Daesh, and the Zionism of the 1940s.

The concept of jihad

There are major differences in understandings of the concept of jihad, as there are with many other ideas that become misused in the service of ideology. Within mainstream Muslim understanding, jihad can be understood as an internal struggle against one's ego and selfishness; this is referred to as "major jihad" in classical Islamic texts. The duty to defend people against oppression or act in self-defense is known as the "minor jihad." The Qur'an states: "And what is [the matter] with you that you fight not in the cause of Allah and [for] the oppressed among men, women, and children who say, 'Our Lord, take us out of this city of oppressive people and appoint for us from Yourself a protector and appoint for us from Yourself a helper?'" (4:75)

The Salafi jihadi perspective departs from these mainstream Muslim concepts. While Al-Qaeda took pains to manipulate Qur'anic scripture to legitimize its terrorism as jihad, Daesh does not even bother to provide such justification.

However, the main understanding of relationships with "the other" in Islam comes from the Qur'an: "Allah does not forbid you from dealing kindly and fairly with those who have neither fought nor driven you out of your homes. Surely Allah loves those who are fair." (60:8) On such a basis, influential Islamic thinkers such as Shaikh Yusuf Al-Qaradawi, Malek Bennabi and Rached

Ghannouchi have affirmed that pluralism, democracy and Islam are not incompatible. The traditional notion of Islamic jihad does not imply a conflict with democracy.

Conflating legitimate Palestinian resistance with transnational jihadism

Conflating legitimate Palestinian resistance with transnational jihadi groups is a common objective of multiple actors, each activated by different motives: Israel's goal, for example, is to recruit further Western support of its occupation of Palestine and to portray itself in the US and Europe as the victim of terror attacks, and thus an expert in fighting "terrorism" whereby it exports military and security expertise to the world.

In Egypt, unfounded claims that Hamas cooperated with jihadi groups in Sinai were exploited to incriminate political opponents, namely the Muslim Brotherhood. Even the Palestinian Authority took to smearing Hamas with a #Hamas=Daesh campaign to incite people against the PA's political opponents.

Israel's claims

Israel never misses an opportunity to link legitimate Palestinian resistance to its military occupation to jihadism and global terrorism, even when such links are patently false. In January 2017, for example, Israeli police officers shot and killed educator Yaqoub Abu Al-Qiyan and injured several others during a demolition programme in the Bedouin village of Umm Al-Hiran. The Israeli media manufactured a story depicting Abu Al-Qiyan as a Daesh activist who struck a policeman with his vehicle; this contradicted all eyewitness accounts, which reported that he had left his house in order to avoid witnessing it being demolished. Only later was a video released exposing the Israeli fabrication; the ramming took place because Abu Al-Qiyan lost control of the vehicle after he had been shot.

In a 2014 speech at the UN, Israeli Prime Minister Benjamin Netanyahu declared, "Hamas is ISIS and ISIS is Hamas." He made this claim even though these two organizations are very different to the point of antagonism in doctrine, jurisdiction and practice. In that same year, a report from the UN Disengagement Observer Force (UNDOF) revealed that Israel has been collaborating with Salafi jihadi groups in the occupied Syrian Golan Heights; this collaboration was not restricted to offering medical aid to the injured members of Jabhat Al-Nusra. On the contrary, reports described the transfer of unspecified supplies from Israel to the Syrians, as well as incidents when Israeli soldiers allowed free passage to Syrians who were not injured.

Yet more striking in its implications is the fact that in April 2017, Moshe Ya'alon, a former Israeli Defence Minister, pointed to a possible collaboration with ISIS. "Firing comes occasionally from regions under the control of the Syrian regime," he explained. "But, once the firing came from ISIS positions—and it immediately apologised." Nobody apologises to a supposed enemy, so we are left wondering whether Daesh views Israel as its friend.

Trans-jihadist discourse on Palestine

Groups such as Al-Qaeda and Daesh which use violations in human rights in the name of Islam are also generous in using Palestine in their rhetoric. Rather than a genuine solidarity, they invoke it because of the legitimacy of the Palestinian cause and its popularity among those targeted by the propaganda for trans-national jihad.

According to Lawrence Wright's account of the rise of Osama Bin Laden, his mother observed that Osama had stopped watching Western films by the time he was 14. She described him as concerned, sad and frustrated by the situation in Palestine, with tears streaming down his face as he watched TV and news reports from the occupied land.

Thomas Hegghammer and Joas Wagemakers, authors of a 2013 study on "The Palestine Effect in the Transnational Jihad Movement", found that Palestinians are not over-represented in Al-Qaeda at either the leadership level or as followers. Only one out of three prominent Palestinian jihadist ideologues therein is focused on Palestine: Abdullah Yusuf Azzam. The others, Al-Maqdisi and Al Falastini, consider Palestinian nationalism antagonistic to the objective of establishing an Islamic state. In the founding declaration of "The Islamic Front for Jihad against the Jews and the Crusaders" (February 1998), Palestine was mentioned only as the third issue justifying transnational jihad against Americans, after the US military presence in Saudi Arabia and the sanctions against Iraq. The statement suggests a religious rather than a humanist interest in Palestine: "If the goals of the Americans in these [Middle Eastern] wars are religious and economic, then it is serving the interest of the Jewish state, and to distract attention from its occupation of Bayt al-Maqdis, [an Arabic name for Jerusalem] and its killing of Muslims there."

Palestine is only one among several issues put forward to convince Muslims to join the jihad, usually stirred up by well-publicized atrocities and political tension in the occupied Palestinian territories. The

Palestinian cause was mentioned not only to lament Israeli oppression but to criticize Palestinian politics, especially when Hamas decided to participate in the 2006 elections. For example, in that year, Al-Qaeda's Ayman Al-Zawahiri said, "Palestine is under occupation and its constitution is man-made and pagan, and Islam has nothing to do with it." This was his way of criticizing Hamas for taking part in the elections. In March 2007, he repeated his criticism, stating, "The Hamas leadership has sold out Palestine, and earlier it had sold out referring to Sharia as the source of jurisdiction."

Further jihadi quotations indicating how the Palestinian cause has been used

"The American people have given their consent to the incarceration of the Palestinian people, the demolition of Palestinian homes and the slaughter of the children of Iraq. This is why the American people are not innocent. The American people are active members in all these crimes." Osama Bin Laden, 14 October 2002

"Has Shaikh Osama Bin Laden not informed you that you will not dream of security until we live it in reality in Palestine?" Ayman Al Zawahiri, 4 August 2005

"Jihad in Palestine and Iraq today is a duty for the people of the two countries and other Muslims." Osama Bin Laden, December 2004

In April 2007, Islamic State of Iraq leader Abu Omar Al-Baghdadi stated that the conflict in Iraq has "paved the way for invading the Jewish state and the restoration of Jerusalem."

Palestine in the Daesh discourse

Daesh has a less elaborate discourse on Palestine than Al-Qaeda. It often uses images depicting Al-Aqsa and the Dome of the

Rock Mosques in its propaganda videos, especially in a context of growing assertions among a pro-regime false intellectual elite in various Arab countries who raise doubts about the Muslim claim to Jerusalem. Daesh also dignifies some leaders with pseudonyms suggesting ties to Jerusalem and Palestine.

Amedy Coulibaly, the gunman who attacked a kosher store in Paris in 2015, is reported by French BFM-TV journalist Sarah-Lou Cohen that he had deliberately chosen to target Jews "to defend oppressed Muslims, notably in Palestine."

In October 2015, Daesh issued videos embracing knife attacks and making suggestions to Palestinians about how to carry them out more effectively. Like the Israelis, the group also makes false claims about lone-wolf attacks by adolescent Palestinians, against all available evidence. As with Al-Qaeda, Daesh attacks the Palestinians' framing of their cause: "Your struggle is not about land, but about right versus wrong. It's about religion." Daesh videos show ritual burning of the Palestinian flag and have been merciless with Palestinian refugees in Syria. The group's reaction to Donald Trump's decision to move the US Embassy to Jerusalem came late and was irrelevant. In an editorial that appeared in *Al-Naba* newsletter, it made use of the occasion to blame other Islamist groups for their "hypocritical and self-serving statements."

The universal dimension of the Palestinian cause
British historian Arnold Toynbee once said, "The tragedy in Palestine is not just a local one; it is a tragedy for the world, because it is an injustice that is a menace to the world's peace." The Palestinian cause has universal echoes, not only because of the

religious value of the Holy Land, but also because Palestine is the location of a current, concrete, protracted area of friction between the dominant, imperialistic West and the Orient. The power relationship manifested in Israel's military occupation of Palestine is an important part of the psychological and social make-up of many people around the world, and the symbolic meaning of Palestinian resistance to the occupation has the potential to liberate many people from their immediate oppression at home.

In the context of this global awareness, it is perhaps inevitable that there has always been a dangerous and violent misrepresentation of the Palestinian plight, from that put forward by the Japanese Red Army (1970) to jihadi groups.

The Palestinian and Arab reaction to jihadist claims

Global jihadi groups have contributed nothing whatsoever to the legitimate Palestinian resistance against Israel's occupation. The reason for this is that Palestinian grievances, narrative and resistance are wholly human, grounded in universally recognized human rights, and emerge from a brutal political reality, not from a perceived promise by God.

It is not surprising that jihadi groups receive little popular support in Palestine and among Arabs generally. Palestinians do not share their political ideology and do not imitate their tactics, since these entail severe human rights violations. A public opinion poll conducted in the West Bank and the Gaza Strip in 2015 by the Palestinian Centre for Policy and Survey Research (PSR) demonstrated that an overwhelming majority (91%) believes that Daesh is a radical group that does not represent true Islam. In 2018, Arab Opinion Index conducted by the Arab Centre for Research and Policy Studies in Qatar revealed the following: Almost all respondents (98%) indicated that they were aware of the "Islamic State" and an overwhelming majority (92%) had a negative view of it, with 2% expressing a "positive" view. Interestingly, among the favourable views, answers were not correlated with religion; respondents who identified themselves as "Not religious" were just as likely to have favourable views of Daesh as those who identified as "Very religious". The researchers concluded that public attitudes toward Daesh are generated by present-day political considerations and not motivated by religion.

When asked for conjecture about the factors which might drive citizens of Arab countries to join Daesh, 42% said political instability in their home countries; 24% said economic conditions; and 6% cited social circumstances such as inequality, marginalization and social exclusion. A further 18% credited "brainwashing" and "propaganda", while a final 6% described the chance to fight foreign powers and/or sectarian militias in Syria and Iraq. Just under 30% of respondents believed that the group's existence resulted from the internal conflicts extant in the Middle East, compared to 59% who attributed it to the policies of foreign powers. When asked to suggest the best means by which to combat Daesh, resolving the Palestinian conflict ranked third among five most commonly reported answers: military means (18%), ending foreign intervention in Arab countries (17%), resolving the Palestinian conflict (13%), supporting democratic transitions (12%) and solving economic issues (9%).

In early 2018, Daesh issued a 22-minute video in which it launched a war on Hamas and described its fighters as "apostates." At the end of the video, Daesh fighter Hamza Zamli ordered a masked man to execute a kneeling Hamas captive, Musa Abu Zamt. The video exposed the ferocious enmity between Daesh and Hamas; the former has been understood generally by the Palestinian public as but another tool to crack down against the Palestinian resistance.

Hamas also distances itself from Salafi jihadists. After a Salafi suicide bomber killed Nidal Ja'afri, a member of the Hamas military wing, on the border with Egypt in August 2017, the resistance movement called Salafi-jihadist views "a perverted ideology" and "a foreign implant." Hamas believes that it is facing at least two adversaries, Israel and Salafi jihadists, with the latter trying "to shift the compass of holy jihad against the Zionist occupiers." The so-called Islamic State accused Hamas of abandoning the Islamic path, capitulating to tyranny, and focusing exclusively on the Gaza Strip, thus abandoning the rest of Palestine. It has even gone as far as calling on its supporters to act against Hamas and its people, a statement backed by the organization's Sinai-based Mufti, Qazem Al-Azawi.

Commonalities between the "Jewish state" and "Islamic State"

Palestinians might be expected to be most repulsed by Daesh because of the similarity in objectives and methods used by the group and the Jewish state established in 1948. I made this comparison in a previous article—"In the aftermath of Paris, the Israeli way is not the answer" in which I argued, "Both Daesh and the 'Jewish state' were established through horrible massacres leaving a population of refugees in their wake. Both display expansionist ambitions. The strategy of Daesh is to attack the West, with the goal of provoking further discrimination against Western Muslims to get them out of the 'grey zone'; Israel's Mossad was behind terror attacks against Jews in Iraq, Egypt and Morocco intended to induce them to move to Israel. Similar is Operation Sushana, in which Israeli spies planned bombing attacks against Egyptian Jews; the deliberate and sustained attack by Israeli aircraft and motor torpedo boats against the USS *Liberty*, killing 34 crew members and wounding 171 others and various false-flag operations around the world are further examples of heinous crimes committed by Israelis for which blame was pinned elsewhere."

And yet, Salafi jihadists share with today's Zionists the delegitimization of the Palestinian nationalist narrative as well as the targeting of Palestinian resistance fighters. Both advocate religious supremacy over fundamental values of society, the principles of democracy and universal human rights. One important difference between the leaders of Zionist terrorism and the men of Daesh is that the former became statesmen and some were awarded the Nobel Peace Prize, while the latter are condemned to death universally.

Tackling the psychological and the contextual

Commitment to Salafi jihadism is an individual process of developing extremist beliefs, emotions and behaviour, but it does not only develop in the mind; it is also influenced by a socio-political context. Research and interventions are so far focused on the "mind of the jihadis." Discrimination, socioeconomic crises, political repression and blocking the way for political and social change through non-violent means all shake people's beliefs in human rights and democracy. These pressures create an opening for certain vulnerable and receptive individuals to engage in binary, absolutistic thinking and perceived in-group superiority. These cognitive distortions serve to resolve their personal feelings of uncertainty, absence of meaning, lack of focus in life and a subjective sense of a fragmented worldview.

We cannot underestimate the effect of the attack on moderate Islamic political organizations such as the Muslim Brotherhood in understanding the radicalization of certain individuals among Muslim youth. It is at such moments of maximum vulnerability that Salafi jihadism appeals to people deprived of their identity to offer a "different solution." Group identification solves the problem of uncertainty and self-doubt (Tajfel, 1979).

Like a few other Western countries that also support oppressive Arab regimes and demonize moderate Islamic groups, France is making efforts to delegitimize efforts to challenge Zionism ideologically. Two months after getting sworn into office, French President Emmanuel Macron declared, "We will not give in to anti-Zionism because it is the reinvented form of anti-Semitism." Last February, Macron said that he was considering pushing forward legislation that equates anti-Zionism with the crime of anti-Semitism. Prime Minister Manuel Valls added, "There is, in the very heart of Islam, this disease that devours Islam, which is anti-Semitism, the hatred of Israel."

France has also used the Lellouche Law, which bans "discrimination" based on national origin, to restrain the BDS movement, a Palestinian-led, international civil society campaign to end international support for Israel's oppression of Palestinians and to pressure the state to comply with international law. Last January, Paul Furia, a spokesman for the French Foreign Ministry, said, "Calling [for a] boycott of Israel is indeed illegal in France." Several decisions of the highest criminal court (the Court of Cassation) confirmed that calling for such a boycott breaks the law and constitutes an incitement to discrimination or hate based on national origin or religion. This, though, was not the position of the French government on the boycott of Russia over its action in Ukraine.

Like the exclusion of Islamists from political life in the Arab world, delegitimizing solidarity with Palestine in France and spreading Islamophobia threaten to push people towards radicalism, playing into the hands of jihadi groups. Jihadist ideologue Abu Musab Al-Suri's 2005 manifesto *The Call to Global Islamic Resistance* argued that conducting attacks on European soil—the "soft underbelly of the West"—would reveal rightist politics there and convince European Muslims that coexistence is not possible in a racist, xenophobic continent.

The moral responsibility of Palestinians

Individuals involved in the Palestinian resistance have a different psychological profile to transnational jihadists: unlike many among the latter, they are not ex-felons, nor are they motivated by supremacy theories, dichotomous thinking or alleged promises from God. The Palestinian resistance accepts democracy, pluralism, political accountability and the concept of the civil state. In occupied Palestine, legitimate resistance strives to hold accountable those responsible for their political oppression, not to harm innocent third parties. It aims to minimize occasions for offence, put forth a modest reaction to attacks initiated against them, and seek opportunities for problem solving and truces. Hamas has neither targeted nor called for targeting any entity other than the Israeli occupation. It has intervened to stop any aggression against foreigners, as in the kidnapping of British journalist Alan Johnston, and has not boasted about the treatment of Israeli prisoners, such as Gilad Shalit.

Palestinians have the moral responsibility to be concerned about how their cause is being used by those outside Palestine. Events in Palestine have stimulated a solidarity-based sense of grievance in non-Palestinians that inspires them to be agents of change. Palestinians have invented avenues and opportunities for global resistance to Zionism and solidarity with Palestinians that do not conflict with either universal human rights or the culture of democracy as stipulated by the Council of Europe in 2016. Some of these resistance movements are BDS, We Are All Mary, and the Global Mental Health Networks.

The people of Palestine can provide a conceptual clarification and an alternative international activism that challenges unjust decisions through peaceful civil engagement. This activism embraces political decisions that prevent violent radicalization and achieve genuine acceptance of the self and the other; it increases rather than diminishes the sense of belonging to a larger human group of socially and morally responsible citizens.

Brunel University Has Buckled Under Pro-Israel Pressure To Silence Palestinian Voices

Originally published on *Middle East Monitor*, 26 April 2022

Earlier this month, Professor Paul Hellewell, Vice Provost and Dean of the College of Health, Medicine and Life Sciences at Britain's Brunel University, assured its students that an "anti-Israel" article recommended as part of a course curriculum would not be used again. The article in question was my 2019 interview published in *Quartz*, which took issue with the applicability of PTSD diagnosis to Palestinian victims of political violence.

Apparently, the objection to my article was first raised by Brunel first-year students in Occupational Therapy and then supported by an organization unrelated to the university, UK Lawyers for Israel (UKLFI). This organization's webpage very clearly identifies its objective as the generation of political messaging in support of the state of Israel. Nevertheless, seemingly without recognizing the irony of its position, UKLFI objected to the use of my published interview as an example of cultural perspectives on medical diagnosis by proclaiming that it is "undesirable to mix the objective study of occupational therapy with political propaganda."

UKLFI claimed that the article was liable to promote hostility towards Jewish students and said: "Emphasising suffering of Palestinians without any reference to suffering of Israelis who are also traumatised by the conflict, the article included misleading and irrelevant allegations against Israel. For example, the article referred to house demolitions in East Jerusalem in a way which implied that they are frequent, when they are extremely rare, and falsely claimed that nearly every Palestinian building is deemed illegal by Israeli authorities."

With regard to these UKFLI claims, it appears that open debate regarding the relevant facts is sorely needed. The 2019 report from the UN Office for the Coordination of Humanitarian Affairs (OCHA) makes clear that only 13% of Israeli-occupied East Jerusalem is zoned for Palestinian construction, whereas 35% is allocated for illegal Israeli settlement; and at least one third of Palestinian homes lack an Israeli permit, potentially placing 100,000 Palestinian at risk of displacement.

Initially, it appeared that open debate at Brunel might be permitted. Under the first UKFLI assault on Brunel's academic freedom, Hellewell apparently did not agree to remove my interview but instead acknowledged that some curriculum materials have the potential to cause distress to students. The UKFLI website explained in February 2022 that Brunel would welcome the opportunity to explore these issues in an open forum. Sadly, however, by this month, Brunel had buckled under pressure and reversed its position. The possibility of open debate was silenced. My interview was stricken from the curriculum.

The case of Brunel University backing down under overtly political, pro-Israel lobby pressure is not new or unique. It is just one example of the hypocrisy, reluctance and ambivalence within academia and elsewhere when it comes to academic freedom and progressive thought generally, especially relating to occupied Palestine.

For Palestinians and other oppressed and colonized peoples, knowledge is the pathway to changing the often dismal reality for the better. However, the obstacles facing us in generating professional knowledge are endless. In my case, I am continuously overworked and robbed of time to reflect on my own experience as a colonial subject, to question and to resist the imprint of coloniality on my thinking and practice. Every contribution is made under the stress of time restriction, sleep deprivation and anxiety about a potential attack and rejection.

There is an ever-present awareness that putting forward an academic contribution is financially draining; conferences and journals ask for fees that can exceed the monthly salary of a specialist Palestinian doctor. How can we share our perspectives with global readers and conference participants when they only represent those who can afford to pay for the conferences and journals to which we try to contribute? The entire process of mainstreaming knowledge overlooks the colonized and oppressed. And when a few Palestinian academics do manage to bypass the obstacles presented by the process, then we also have to face intimidation and exclusion by Israel and its supporters. The influence of pro-Israel lobby groups such as UKLFI and the Canary Mission website in the silencing of Palestinian voices is pervasive.

At this time, the ongoing and long-term professional hypocrisy regarding Palestine is being exposed through the willingness to discuss Ukraine within the spheres of academia, mental health and sports. Brunel University has missed an opportunity to resist the pressure for "Palestinian exception" and to welcome a full range of intellectual perspectives, including decolonial thought. Instead, the university has fallen prey to pro-Israel lobbying and thus contributes to the repression and silencing of the trauma in occupied Palestine.

Arab Normalisation Is Another Attempt To Defeat The Palestinians Psychologically

Originally published on *Middle East Monitor*, 24 September 2020

Last week, Israeli Prime Minister Benjamin Netanyahu and foreign ministers representing the United Arab Emirates and Bahrain signed the "Abraham Accords Peace Agreement" in Washington DC which normalizes their relations at the expense of Palestinian national and human rights. US President Donald Trump hosted the ceremony and has claimed that these deals are just the beginning and that there will be other countries making similar agreements very soon, ending Israel's isolation in the region and thereby excluding the Palestinians.

The Arab League refused to back the Palestinians and voted down a resolution denouncing the normalization deals. Earlier, Jared Kushner, Trump's senior advisor and son-in-law, had toured the Middle East to meet with Arab leaders, even those in post-revolution Sudan, which had been promised an end to sanctions and removal from the list of terrorist states if it follows in the UAE's footsteps. By seeking to buy more friends in support of the Israeli occupation and boost his record of achievements, Kushner hopes to deliver more votes to "Trump the peace broker" just in time for the US presidential election in November, all at the expense of the Palestinians.

In order to reduce the cognitive dissonance for the Arab masses, this political process has been synchronized with a public relations and social media campaign promoting a "fascination with Israel."

Supporting this effort is the broadcast of stories and films in Arabic celebrating the humanity, beauty and progressive nature of Israel. This discourse completely deletes the Palestinian narrative and the undisputable suffering of the people over many decades. Indeed, it is a campaign that smears the reputation of the people of Palestine, denies Israel's brutal occupation and asserts that Palestinians willingly sold their lands and homes to the Zionist state. This fake narrative asserts that the Palestinians and their complaints are a drain on the Arab world and promotes the hashtag #Palestine is not my cause. All of this is taking place while Israel is demolishing Palestinian homes, killing unarmed Palestinian civilians and arresting Palestinian children in the midst of both normalization with Arab states and the Covid-19 pandemic.

All Palestinian political parties have condemned the US-brokered accords as a "stab in the back." The Palestinian Prime Minister described them as "black day in the sad calendar" of Palestinian history. They are indeed another attempt to defeat the Palestinians psychologically.

The Palestinian people are undoubtedly outraged by the normalizing Arab states and the helplessness of their own representatives. I've seen Palestinians weeping in the streets at seeing the flags of the normalization countries projected on the walls of Jerusalem. They view the deals as a treacherous betrayal of the Palestinian cause and a belittling of Palestinian and Arab sacrifices over many decades.

I understand that the Palestinian Authority is not against normalization in principle, but is, rather, against a process of "normalization" that excludes them as participants. It is one of the ironies of the current process that the Palestinian representatives during the Oslo years have paved the way for Arab leaders to move towards their own normalization with Israel. Moreover, the PA apprehends that the current normalization prepares the way for Mohammed Dahlan to replace his adversary Mahmoud Abbas as PA President, being a loyal ally of the US, the UAE and Israel.

The official call for a "day of rage" on 15 September was not observed by many Palestinians, since many people are fatigued by political hypocrisy and doubt that public mobilization has much impact on the regional and international world order. Over the Oslo decades, Palestinian representatives—through both conscious and unconscious motivations of their own—have weakened community resilience within Palestine substantially. Legitimate Palestinian resistance was undermined by the absence of democratic processes. Now the Palestinian representatives appear to have recognized that they are powerless within international politics and, as a result, are attempting to revive a Palestinian revolutionary discourse as a means of hiding behind the spirit of the ordinary people.

The very name "Abraham Accords" is misleading and masks the colonial nature of Israel's occupation of Palestine. By presenting it as a religious conflict between the "Abrahamic faiths" Israel erases the political rights of the Palestinians; the occupation is hidden beneath the notion that conflict resolution is about interfaith understanding. The reality is that the enemies of democracy and human rights in the Arab world are realigning themselves in a coalition that tramples Palestinian rights. In doing so, they are destroying the Palestinians' future by withdrawing support from within the Arab world. This process undermines the cultural connection between Palestine and the larger geographical and historical context. Palestinians already feel like orphans; the new normalization only adds to their sense of abandonment by the bigger "Arab brothers."

The ongoing discussion involving yet more Arab countries preparing to announce normalization with Israel is even more damaging and confusing for Palestine. The Palestinian experience has some parallels with a woman enduring a mass sexual assault; that the crime is done under the protective cover of the group makes the experience even more psychologically damaging.

Nevertheless, let Israel toast its new friends among Arab dictators and enjoy the blessings of the Arab League in the knowledge that these "representatives" do not actually represent anyone, least of all the Arab people. The masses, in fact, remain loyal to Palestine, but are exploited by their regimes willing to betray both them and Palestine in return for political and military support from Israel and the US.

When all is said and done, Israel must still deal with Palestinians resisting the occupation at the nominal border fence surrounding the Gaza Strip; at the Dheisheh Refugee Camp in the occupied West Bank; among the Eisaweyeh Jerusalemites; and with others who remain undefeated psychologically. These people and places will remind the Israelis of their unfinished business with Palestinians and the decades of their exploitation of the people and the land. Palestinians have been fighting for their national and human rights for generations and will continue to do so. In a struggle which now takes the shape of a US–European-backed but Israeli-led invasion of the Arab world, Palestine remains on the front line in the struggle for justice.

Sculpting Liberation: Tales of Marco Cavallo and the Jenin Battle Horse

Originally published in Italian, 27 March 2024

Within the tales of resilience and resistance, many remarkable symbols have emerged; to me, two of these symbols have been statues of horses—one sculpture named Marco Cavallo and the other known as Al-Hissan, the Jenin Battle Horse. Their stories weave together the threads of art, symbolism, and an intricate mix of social and political factors shaping mental health. The tales of these two statues offer profound insights into the universal human need for expression and the unique challenges faced by people living under oppression.

Imagine yourself within the walls of Trieste's San Giovanni asylum, where the sculpture called Marco Cavallo stands tall, a beacon of hope amid adversity. Born in 1973 through the collaborative efforts of patients, artists and staff, this majestic blue horse symbolizes the transformative journey of deinstitutionalization that swept through Italy's psychiatric services. Under the guidance of the visionary Franco Basaglia, the asylum's director, the Marco Cavallo statue became more than just a sculpture; it became a testament to the healing power of art and community within mental healthcare. Named after its equine predecessor, Marco the horse, this sculpture embodies the longing for freedom and dignity within the confines of the asylum, marking a profound shift towards reconnecting the domain of the asylum with the outside world.

Now, shift your gaze to the ravaged streets of Jenin, where the Palestinian community witnessed the birth of another symbol:

the Jenin Battle Horse. Standing tall amidst the debris of conflict, this 16-foot sculpture, crafted from the metal remnants of ambulances, became a beacon of resilience and defiance. Designed by the German artist Thomas Kilpper in collaboration with the children of Jenin—children who bore witness to the horrors of the 2002 massacre—Al-Hissan embodied the capacity of the human spirit's ability to rise above tragedy. Yet, in a cruel twist of fate, the Israeli military targeted this symbolic horse, seeking to erase not only its physical presence but also the memory of Palestinian strength and identity that this work of art represented. The statue was destroyed.

The contrasting fates of Marco Cavallo and Al-Hissan highlight the struggles faced by Palestinians as they grapple with loss and oppression. While Marco Cavallo symbolizes liberation within the asylum's walls, Al-Hissan's destruction reflects the ongoing battle against settler violence and the Israeli attempt to erase Palestinian history and identity.

Symbols hold a deep psychological significance, especially in the face of adversity. They become vessels for suppressed narratives and assertions of identity, serving as powerful forms of resistance against erasure. In Palestine, where political factors heavily influence mental health, art and symbolism emerge as vital tools for expression and healing, calling for culturally sensitive and contextually relevant interventions.

From a human perspective, both Marco Cavallo and Al-Hissan are vehicles for the innate human need for symbolism and collective memory in times of trauma. While Marco Cavallo signifies progress and empowerment in mental healthcare, Al-Hissan's destruction reflects the ongoing trauma endured by Palestinian communities.

Yet a symbol cannot be exterminated. The stories of Marco Cavallo and the Jenin Battle Horse offer profound insights into the resilience of the human spirit and the power of collective memory. They remind us of the critical role symbols play in mental health and highlight the urgent need for comprehensive support of communities affected by conflict and oppression. As we reflect on their tales, we are reminded of the enduring significance of symbols in the fight for freedom and justice, and the profound impact they hold for oppressed communities worldwide.

Cultivating Resilience: A Palestinian recipe for the well-being of activists

Originally published in *Activist Wellbeing Cookbook*, 29 January 2024

For activists and the defenders of freedom working and living in regions besieged by occupation, colonization, and oppression, the psychological toll can be immense. The relentless exposure to violence, loss, and trauma can lead to profound psychological challenges, including anxiety, depression, traumatic stress, emotional fatigue, and burnout.

The psyches of activists are continually bombarded with information, images, and memories that disrupt their peace of mind, creating a feeling of pain and moral injury. When they escape direct threat or retaliation, witnessing horrible actions that violate one's ethical beliefs can cause profound helplessness, guilt, shame, confusion, and a crisis of identity. For those fighting for justice, the moral conflict between necessary actions and deeply held values can be particularly tormenting. Among activists are those who survive when others do not—and who therefore often grapple with survivor's guilt, questioning why they lived while others perished, making it difficult to find peace or feel deserving of life's small joys.

Sumud: The essence of Palestinian resilience

In the context of the Palestinian struggle, the concept of Sumud—steadfastness or perseverance—embodies the spirit of our resistance. Sumud is not just about enduring hardship; it is about maintaining our identity, dignity, defiance to oppression, and hope for freedom in the face of relentless oppression.

Sumud can apply to the mental health and well-being of those who resist state repression and fight for liberation around the world. It teaches us to stand firm, to draw strength from our roots, and to believe in the possibility of a just future. Sumud is about finding strength in community, in our shared struggles, and in the unyielding belief that justice will prevail.

For activists, embracing Sumud means cultivating resilience, fostering solidarity, and nurturing hope. It is the promise to not give up, even in weak moments, until we find the power to stand up again to our cause and to continue the fight for a better world. Through Sumud, we honor the past, live fully in the present, and remain committed to a future of freedom and justice.

My personal perspective

As a psychiatrist in Palestine, keeping myself afloat amid pervasive trauma and ongoing violence is a complex but deeply rooted process. I was born into a traumatic context, so that my defenses and survival mechanisms have developed naturally and steadily over my life. These mechanisms are not just my personal way of survival; they are a testament to the Sumud that defines me as a Palestinian.

On a more specific level, my faith plays a central role in my life. I sense Allah's care and mercy guiding me through the most challenging times. This faith not only provides me with strength and solace but also instills in me a sense of purpose and duty. I firmly believe that the Palestinian cause is a just and noble human cause that I am honored to defend; I think I would have done the same if I were not a Palestinian. I think it is a profound example of a confrontation between right and might, which is a common reality that can be experienced everywhere. In this struggle, the example is

Palestinian, but the lesson is global. This belief provokes my sense of responsibility and ignites my perseverance and determination. My supportive family and reliable friends are a cornerstone of my strength. They provide me with a network of emotional support, understanding, and encouragement, which is essential in the face of ongoing adversity. We share a common bond and understanding of our struggles, which reinforces our collective steadfastness.

For me, my profession is not just a job; it is a calling that allows me to be of service to my community. By helping others heal, I find purpose and avoid becoming paralyzed by the traumatic help-lessness meant to be inflicted upon us in Palestine. This active engagement in the healing process reinforces my engagement and sense of agency.

Ultimately, I do what I believe I have to do in my life, guided by a deep sense of purpose and acceptance of consequences. This acceptance brings me comfort, even in the midst of turmoil. By integrating my faith, the support of family and friends, and my professional purpose, I navigate the immense challenges of my work and life in Palestine with a resilient heart and a hopeful spirit. I understand that Palestine is in difficult and painful labor, and our liberation will come one day.

Of course, there are many difficult times. When I feel tired, sad, or grieving, I especially find peace in my connection to the land.

My journey towards healing amid the pervasive trauma of occupation has led me to the humble yet profound practice of gardening. The sanctuary of flickering leaves and blooming flowers became my refuge, offering a respite from the haunting accounts of torture and suffering that I encountered daily in my profession. Gardening videos initially helped me push out the residual images of horror and flashbacks, and once I moved to a house with an allotment, I embraced the practice wholeheartedly, and started planting my organic vegetables and fruits.

In the aftermath of the heart-wrenching losses inflicted by the genocide in Palestine, gardening became more than a hobby—it became a lifeline, a sacred ritual through which I communed with the land and honored the souls of those who had fallen. Amid a brutal political strategy aimed at weaponizing starvation, planting my own food was a profound act of defiance. The occupying forces sought to starve our people into submission; every seed I planted was a rebellion against this oppressive tactic, a declaration of a Palestinian will to live, to nourish ourselves, and to resist.

Each seed planted was a whispered prayer for the departed, each blossom a tribute to their enduring spirit. The garden became a microcosm of Sumud and resistance. Every vegetable that sprouted, every fruit that ripened, was a testament to our resilience. Nothing went to waste—food scraps were turned into compost, enriching the soil that, in turn, sustained us. This cycle of growth and renewal was a powerful counter-narrative to the destruction and despair imposed upon us.

As I worked the soil with my hands, I felt a profound connection to the earth beneath me—a connection that transcended mere physicality and touched upon the very essence of existence. In the fertile soil, I saw the precious bodies of martyrs interwoven with the roots of the plants, their souls mingling with the fragrant blossoms that adorned the garden.

Every morning, as the first light of dawn kissed the horizon, I would walk among the rows of vegetables and flowers, tenderly nurturing each plant as if it were a cherished soul. And as the sun dipped below the horizon, I would offer my gratitude to the land that had become my safe haven, my shrine, and my companion in grief.

My garden is a reminder that even in the darkest of times, life finds a way to bloom anew—that from the ashes of destruction, beauty can still emerge. Observing the seasons, experiencing loss and death in this natural context, and witnessing new growth provides me with a profound sense of grounding. It reminds me of the continuity of life and the hope inherent in nature.

Other strategies for mental well-being and healing
While I find my mindfulness and meditation in gardening, others might find it in praying, relaxing, contemplating, etc. Techniques such as deep breathing, progressive muscle relaxation, and guided imagery can be beneficial to many people. These practices ground us in the present moment, providing respite from the relentless march of traumatic memories.

For some, building and maintaining strong community ties is essential. Sharing experiences, offering mutual support, and fostering a sense of solidarity can mitigate feelings of isolation and helplessness. Together, activists gain synergy, drawing strength from each other's resilience and shared purpose.

Engaging in creative activities such as writing, art, music, and dance can serve as powerful outlets for processing emotions and expressing the inexpressible. Art transforms pain into beauty, giving voice to the unspoken and renovating a sense of subjectivity and agency.

Sometimes, accessing professional mental health support, such as peer support, therapy or counseling, can provide invaluable assistance. Human rights organizations and solidarity groups should strive to provide access to mental health resources for activists and establish environments where activists feel safe to share their experiences and emotions without judgment. Safe spaces foster open dialogue and containment. Encouraging a culture that prioritizes self-care and mutual support, recognizing that caring for oneself is integral to sustaining the fight for justice, and promoting a culture of care validates the need for rest and recuperation.

It is also important for every activist to recognize one's limits and set boundaries to prevent burnout. Taking regular breaks, delegating tasks, and ensuring time for rest and self-care are critical.

As I reflect on the fruits and vegetables I harvest from my garden, I am reminded of the French proverb, *"chacun fait sa cuisine interne,"* which means "everyone creates his own worldview." This metaphor speaks to the unique blend of ingredients that contribute to our well-being. For activists, it is vital to remember that their personal well-being is essential to sustaining the noble causes they champion. Each of us must find the right balance of practices that nurture our resilience and Sumud, enabling us to continue our fight for justice with vigor and clarity.

Islam And Liberation Psychology: A pillar of psychological struggle in occupied Palestine

Originally published on *Middle East Monitor*, 27 September 2024

Liberation psychology is a revolutionary approach in the field of psychology that goes beyond traditional therapy to focus on addressing the social and political roots of oppression and injustice based on the voices and experiences of the powerless (Heitz, 2022). It is a direct response to the suffering of colonized and oppressed people, with the aim to free the mind and soul from the destructive effects of internalized colonization and occupation. In Palestine, where people live under the burden of occupation, liberation psychology is a pressing necessity to confront injustice and its psychological and social effects. This approach is not limited to individual psychological dimensions but is deeply intertwined with the struggle for freedom and justice in the societies where people live.

In Palestine, Islamic principles emerge as a fundamental pillar that can support and enhance this form of liberation. Islam, embedded with teachings that call for justice, equality, and the rejection and confrontation of oppression, aligns with the goals of liberation psychology in building resistant societies that strive for dignity and liberation from all forms of tyranny. Islam carries within it a comprehensive liberation message that extends to multiple aspects of human life, from the liberation of the soul and psyche to the liberation of society from injustice and tyranny (Dabous, 2018). Liberation is fundamental in Islam and and is founded on the idea of building individuals and communities with values of justice, dignity, and perseverance in the face of oppression. As a psychiatrist, I cannot comprehend the endurance, resilience, and steadfastness of the Palestinian community in the face of all the challenges we experience without recognizing the pivotal role Islam plays in the culture of the society. The glorification of martyrs and the hope of meeting loved ones in the afterlife offer comfort to people enduring loss and grief when the tools of psychiatry and all forms of therapy fall short in alleviating these deep psychological wounds.

Liberation in Islam forms an important foundation for the emergence of a Muslim liberation psychology that focuses on addressing the causes and effects of injustice on mental health. Islam is a religion that elevates the value of human dignity and defends human freedom on all levels. Allah says in the Qur'an: "And We have certainly honored the children of Adam" (Al-Isra: 70). This verse reflects how human dignity is at the core of Islam's message, where it must not be violated under any circumstance. Islam came to liberate humanity from all forms of enslavement, not only physically but also intellectually and psychologically (Kunnumal, 2023).

Liberating the self from psychological constraints and pressures is an integral part of the Islamic message. The Qur'an encourages liberation from fear and dependence on oppressors, urging believers to rely on Allah SWT and trust in themselves. Allah SWT says: "So fear them not, but fear Me, if you are [indeed] believers" (Al-Imran: 175). This verse directs Muslims to rid themselves of the psychological fear that forces of oppression may instill in them, affirming that true fear should be of Allah SWT alone, opening the door to freeing the soul from subjugation.

Muslims consider resisting injustice a religious and moral duty. In Surat An-Nisa, Allah SWT commands the believers to uphold justice and testify to the truth even in the most difficult circumstances: "O you who have believed, be persistently standing firm in justice, witnesses for Allah, even if it be against yourselves" (An-Nisa: 135). This verse places a great responsibility on Muslims to achieve justice and oppose oppression.

Prophet Muhammad (peace be upon him) reinforced this principle in his statement: "The best jihad is a word of truth in front of a tyrannical ruler" (reported by al-Tirmidhi), highlighting that jihad is not only through arms but also by confronting tyranny and oppression with words and taking a stand against injustice, which can be a cornerstone of liberation psychology.

Islam as a revolution against the social structures of pre-Islamic Arabia

In the time of Prophet Muhammad's (PBUH) mission, the Arabian Peninsula was living under rigid and harsh social structures characterized by class discrimination, economic exploitation, racial oppression, and tribal violence. These structures bolstered the authority of the elite and depended on the enslavement and exploitation of the weak. Islam came to overturn these social structures and establish a new society based on justice and equality (Kunnummal, 2023).

The most prominent aspect of the new Islamic order was the dismantling of class and tribal distinctions, as Prophet Muhammad (PBUH) declared in his farewell sermon: "O people, your Lord is one, and your father is one. There is no superiority of an Arab over a non-Arab, nor of a non-Arab over an Arab, nor of a white over a black, nor of a black over a white, except by piety" (reported by Ahmad). This revolutionary proclamation dismantled the discriminatory social structures of pre-Islamic times and laid the foundation for a society based on equality among all people.

Islam also revolted against slavery, making piety and good deeds the true measure of a person's worth, regardless of their lineage or social class. The Qur'an says: "Freeing a slave" (Al-Balad: 13) is one of the deeds that draw a person closer to Allah. This social revolution was not just material liberation but also offered psychological and intellectual liberation, freeing minds and hearts from the shackles of discrimination and oppression.

Contemporary Islamic liberation leaders

The liberation values of Islam were embodied in the lives of many leaders who used Islam as a tool for liberation from injustice and oppression. Here, we mention some leaders from our modern history, who presented different yet complementary models of how to employ Islam in the struggle for freedom and justice.

Malcolm X is one of the most prominent leaders and activists in the civil rights movement in the United States. He was born in 1925 and died in 1965 in New York. Malcolm X grew up in a challenging environment, where his family faced racial persecution after his father was killed in an incident believed to have racist motives, and his mother suffered psychological crises. His life deteriorated, and he became involved in crime and spent time in prison. During his imprisonment, he embraced Islam, began to reshape his life and thinking, and became a prominent symbol of the struggle for Black rights. He was known for his bold and outspoken stance against racism and oppression. He called for pride in Black identity and for the economic and political independence of Black people in the United States. He later adopted a global perspective and began advocating for cooperation between races and for human rights on a broader scale until he was assassinated on 21 February 1965, while giving a speech in New York. Notably, he visited the Khan Younis camp in 1964, wrote an anti-Zionist article, and met with Ahmad Shukeiri, the first president of the Palestine Liberation Organization. Despite his early death, Malcolm X's legacy remained alive, and he is considered today one of the symbols of the struggle for justice and human dignity.

Before him, there was Abdul Rahman al-Kawakibi, the Syrian thinker and reformer, who was one of the pioneers of the Arab Renaissance. Born in the mid-19th century in Aleppo, Syria, Kawakibi came from a prestigious and well-known family. He studied religious sciences, languages, and modern sciences, which helped him become an influential figure in Arab and Islamic thought. Al-Kawakibi was known for his bold stances against tyranny and injustice, especially against the Ottoman despotism that dominated the Arab world at the time. He called for political, social, and religious reform and believed that despotism was the cause of the decline of the Islamic nation. Thus, he focused on critiquing absolute authority and called for the establishment of a free and just society based on the principles of consultation (*shura*) and democracy. His most famous work is the book *The Nature of Tyranny and the Struggle Against Enslavement*, considered one of the most important texts in Arab political thought. In it, he analyzed the nature of tyranny, its negative effects on society, and offered insights on how to confront and eliminate it.

Ali Shariati was an Iranian thinker and reformer, regarded as one of the influential figures in modern Islamic thought. Born in 1933, his father was a religious activist and intellectual, which had a significant impact on Shariati during his early years. He studied sociology at the University of Mashhad in Iran and completed his higher studies at the Sorbonne in Paris, where he was influenced by Western philosophers and thinkers. This exposure helped him develop his own intellectual vision. Shariati was known for his reformist thought, calling for the reinterpretation of Islam in line with contemporary social and political issues. He focused on reviving Islam as a liberation force against injustice and tyranny. He viewed Islam as a religion that promotes social justice and equality. Shariati authored many books and lectures that influenced the younger generation of Iranians, playing a significant role in shaping the revolutionary consciousness that contributed to the Iranian Revolution of 1979. His most famous works include *Return to Self*, *The Creation of a Revolutionary Self*, and *Religion Against Religion*. To this day, Shariati is regarded as a symbol of Islamic intellectual renewal and a proponent of liberating Muslim peoples from tyranny and injustice. In his book *History of Civilization*, Shariati wrote: "When Palestine is erased from existence, and Jerusalem is occupied, and we hear only a few voices from our scholars, all religious narratives and slogans will become a set of words that mean nothing." (Oxford Encyclopedia of the Islamic World)

From South Africa, Farid Esack emerged as an Islamic scholar and human rights activist. He is considered one of the most prominent contemporary Islamic thinkers working at the intersection of religion with social justice and human rights. Born in 1956, Esack lived his youth during the apartheid era in South Africa, which significantly influenced his thinking and political activism. Esack founded the Muslim Justice Movement in South Africa, which worked to combat apartheid from an Islamic perspective, focusing on resisting injustice and oppression. He was also a supporter of women's rights and participated in discussions on religious and intellectual reform in the Muslim world, making him a prominent voice in this field. In addition to his political and social activism, Esack has held academic positions at several universities around the world, including Harvard University, and is known for research that combines Islamic studies with human rights issues, gender equality, and democracy. Through his works and speeches, Esack called for applying the values of justice and human dignity in Muslim society, emphasizing the importance of positive interaction between Islam and global human rights principles. He remains active in advocating for Palestinian rights (Rahemtulla, 2017).

Many Islamic leaders have demonstrated how Islam can be a driving force for liberation from oppression and tyranny. Islam is not just a religion; it is a liberation message that calls for justice, equality, and solidarity with the oppressed. Islamic history is filled with honourable examples of leaders who stood up to tyrants with the strength of faith and the courage of their convictions. Those values are still alive today in the struggles of oppressed peoples. While some are shackled by fear and submission, Islam continues to inspire souls toward liberation and resistance, so that truth remains steadfast and justice remains the highest goal, worthy of all life's sacrifices.

Palestinian Sumud: A gift to a world facing global tyranny

Originally published in French, 15 August 2024

When Gazans endure bombardment, hunger, and the agony of untreated amputations and injuries, they often instinctively find solace in invoking one of Allah's many names. This form of reliance on Allah offers believers sanctuary and stability. One of Allah's names, aṣ-Ṣamad, (the Samad) reflects this reliance—representing a primordial anchor that is sought during difficult trials. While the act of seeking Allah's help is not called Ṣumūd, the Palestinian notion is deeply embedded in the Islamic faith.

Historically, the term Samad was used by Arabs to describe uniquely resilient and dependable leaders and warriors. Invoking Allah's name aṣ-Ṣamad in moments of vulnerability and fear involves recognizing Him as the ultimate refuge. This name appears only once in the Qur'an, in Sūrat al-Ikhlāṣ: "Say, 'He is Allah—the Uniquely One. Allah, aṣ-Ṣamad (the eternally Besought of all). He neither begets nor is born. Nor is there to Him any equivalent'" (Qur'an 112:1-4). Aṣ-Ṣamad (the Samad) signifies Allah's majesty and grandeur, filling believers with awe and reverence. Thus, sumud involves seeking a superior to aid in reaching what one cannot achieve alone. Belief in aṣ-Ṣamad means emptying our hearts of dependence on anything other than Allah, acknowledging that while we may seek help from others, only Allah can truly fulfill all our needs. This belief leads to moral transcendence, rising above worldly desires and threats.

While sumud aligns with many other Islamic values such as

patience, justice, and determination, it is not confined to Islam, it is a profound principle ingrained in Palestinian culture and resistance, transcending religious boundaries. It is a concept encompassing cultural, national, political and social dimensions, embraced by Palestinians of various religious backgrounds, including Muslims, Christians, and atheist individuals, particularly in the context of resisting the occupation. Palestinian sumud signifies steadfastness, resilience, and perseverance in enduring resistance to displacement, oppression, and socio-political challenges. It is not simply an active political or a passive psychological stance but a way of life that involves the dialectic between the two positions, reflecting a deep-seated belief in the right to exist and thrive in one's homeland despite enduring and often harsh challenges.

Sumud has been exemplified throughout Palestinian history since the resistance to the British Mandate. Here are a few recent examples: The Bedouin village of Al-Arakib in the Negev desert, for example, has been demolished numerous times by Israeli authorities, yet the residents repeatedly rebuild their homes. Palestinian farmers in the Jordan Valley face frequent harassment, land confiscation, and water restrictions by Israeli authorities and settlers. Despite these challenges, many farmers continue to cultivate their lands, embodying sumud by sustaining their agricultural heritage and livelihood. In Hebron, Palestinians and international activists established the "Sumud House" in the Tel Rumeida neighborhood, promoting Palestinian presence and resilience in an area with a heavy Israeli settler and military presence. The Al-Kurd family and other Palestinian families in the Sheikh Jarrah neighborhood of East Jerusalem have become symbols of sumud, resisting eviction threats from Israeli settlers and drawing international attention to their plight.

Palestinian students and teachers in the West Bank face obstacles such as checkpoints, travel restrictions, and school demolitions. Despite these barriers, they pursue education as a form of resistance, viewing it as essential for their community's future. Grassroots organizations, known as Popular Committees, organize non-violent protests and activities in villages like Bil'in and Ni'lin, leading weekly demonstrations against the Israeli separation barrier, land confiscations, and settlement expansions. The Gaza Grand March of Return affirming the collective agency of refugees, Palestinian Heritage Festivals, and women empowerment initiatives all highlight the spirit of sumud among Palestinians.

Key aspects of Palestinian sumud include maintaining and preserving Palestinian community, cultural and national identity through holding onto land, heritage, and traditions despite external pressures of deculturization and memoricide. Sumud emphasizes hope, community solidarity, and the will to endure hardships without giving up the dream of self-determination and liberation. It is about mental and emotional determination, activism, and resistance—striving for rights, even symbolically, that assert self and national emancipation. Sumud also involves collective action, strong community ties, solidarity, and containment.

Sumud and psychological resilience share similarities but differ in their contexts and applications. While sumud reflects steadfastness, perseverance, and the ability to endure hardship and adversity, resilience refers to the capacity to recover quickly from stress and trauma, adapt to change, and keep going in the face of adversity. Both concepts involve significant inner strength and mental fortitude, but sumud is deeply rooted in the Palestinian socio-political context, encompassing the collective cultural and national ethos tied to resisting occupation and displacement, and to maintaining identity. Unlike resilience, it is not limited to the realm of self, it includes changing power structures that oppress the self. Sumud involves collective actions within to a national struggle, including physical existence, cultural preservation, and political resistance. Resilience, on the other hand, focuses on individual psychological coping mechanisms, emotional regulation, positive thinking, searching for social support, and engaging in adaptive behavior to overcome challenges. Sumud, encompasses the meaning of psychological resilience, but is not limited to it, as it is intertwined with action for political change.

Supporting the sumud of the Palestinian people requires a multifaceted approach combining awareness, advocacy, economic aid, cultural preservation, and international solidarity efforts. By undertaking these actions, individuals and organizations can contribute to the resilience and perseverance of Palestinians in their struggle for justice and self-determination.

Supporting sumud is not only necessary for decolonizing Palestine and liberating its people from oppression, but it also provides an opportunity for Palestinian decolonial mental health to influence mainstream mental health practices. While Israel engages in the global export of automated mass killing, spying technology, and policing of people, sumud is the Palestinian gift to a world that must to stand up and challenge global tyranny.

About Solidarity

Professional Solidarity With Palestine: A mental health imperative

Originally published on *OpenDemocracy*, 4 December 2018

In the field of medicine, we often speak of the social determinants of health. In Palestine, not only social, but political determinants of health have a grave impact on the well-being and mental health of our community. I am not just talking about the political blackmail through recent blatant cuts of the US administration of millions of US dollars from East Jerusalem hospitals and defunding UNRWA educational and health services, but also through the daily realities of dismal work opportunities, a vacuum of leadership, the threat of political detention haunting our youth, and the pervasive experiences of loss and grief. Centuries of political oppression has created a cascade of damage to collective identity and individuals' personalities.

The ongoing siege of Gaza is only a single dramatization of how the political realities of occupation deliberately destroy the quality of life for Palestinians. In a society where the sudden traumatic death of young people is common and the experience of detention and torture touch every family, psychological suffering and collective anxiety are pandemics. Who better than mental health professionals to understand how this omnipresent pain and fear can intimidate the population or even push individuals into radicalization?

In my governmental office at the mental health unit responsible for mental health services in the West Bank, I often receive donors and representative of international medical and mental health NGOs, who are interested in supporting our mental health system. Some are ready to pay for medications, equipment, training; but they shy away from advocacy and political solidarity.

But solidarity with the Palestinian people and advocacy for their human and national rights is just a therapeutic stand in the face of their collective historical trauma and is not limited to mental health professionals. Without such solidarity, the interventions of mental health professionals may do more harm than good, as such interventions fail to be preventive, might pathologise the experience of Palestinians, medicalizes their reactions and inhibits their agency, while maintaining the status quo of their pathogenic context.

The decision by the International Association for Relational Psychoanalysis and Psychotherapy (IARPP) to hold its 2019 conference in Tel Aviv, and the participation of the Association de Conferences de Psychiatrie de l'Enfant et de l'Adolescent de Langue Francaise en Israel (COPELFI)—at a colloquium on Trauma in Rennes, France, this December—are recent examples of how occupied Palestine is overlooked by mental health professionals, demonstrating how Western identification with the Israeli experience is facilitated. But this bias is classical in my profession; I use search engines often to see how much is published in my professional domain in relation to Palestine and Israel: so little is published about Palestinian trauma, so much is published about Palestinian "terrorism", while so much is published about Israeli trauma, so little is published about Israel's terrorism.

Propaganda is not limited to media! Even in professional settings, Palestine is hushed, and the final considerations of the trauma of the Jewish nation are silencing much of the critical dialogue about the occupation. In 2014, just after the massacres in Gaza, I was invited to speak at the Tavistock and Portman Institute in London. After multiple attempts to intimidate me into silence, one of the professional participants shouted at the moderator, "This is one-sided; why didn't you invite an Israeli speaker?" "It is a betrayal of the Jewish founding fathers of this place to invite a person like her!"—a psychiatrist who raises questions about the role and responsibility that professionals share to engage with the political reality.

Europeans, Westerners, and Israelis do not own the profession of healing, nor do they possess the experience of Palestinians. To disregard the experience of Palestinians is—at the very least—neglect; to condition listening to and inviting Palestinians to inviting Israelis is an illusion of symmetry and a promotion of the Palestinian normalization with, and dependency on, Israelis to reach international professional venues; that ominous dependency that makes the trauma of the Palestinians more complex. Instead of questioning Israeli professionals about their ethical responsibilities as Israelis and as professionals towards the political trauma of Palestinians, international professionals become an accomplice in denial and that impedes their role as a third party with a potential role to promote psychological healing and encourage restorative justice and future reconciliation.

Many professionals today take pride in having maintained solidarity with Nelson Mandela and the people he represented in his opposition to the apartheid regime of South Africa years ago. Few today would wish to be known as having brought pro-apartheid white South African professionals to conferences so that they could share the expertise of their trauma caused by black South

Africans. Likewise, mental health professionals should not depend upon Israelis to provide expertise on the shock of our political reality. Instead, mental health professionals should take pride in supporting their colleagues in Palestine in their daily work and in generating knowledge and awareness of the human rights abuses perpetrated by the state of Israel that engendered trauma for both peoples. Meanwhile, we, Palestinian mental health professionals, will continue our critical dialogue of the occupation until its hegemony is exposed and deconstructed.

The Thinking Behind The Mental Health Workers' Pledge

Originally published on *UK Palestine Mental Health Network*, 12 November 2015

The Israeli occupation of Palestine

In a time of global turmoil surrounding refugee crises in many areas, it is easy to lose sight of the fact that the Palestinians compose one of the largest refugee populations as well as the most longstanding refugee population in the world. Of the 11.6 million Palestinians dispersed worldwide, 4.5 million individuals live today in stateless insecurity within the Israeli-dominated Occupied Palestinian Territory, a geographically discontinuous, increasingly fragmented, and ever-shrinking area including the West Bank, East Jerusalem, and Gaza. The displacement of the Palestinians from their homes by Israeli forces, beginning in 1948 and continuing through the present moment, is fundamentally a consequence of a single factor: the Israeli ambition to clear the land for its exclusive use by Jewish/Israeli people. The catastrophic impact of this ambition has been endured by generations of Palestinians who have suffered the devastating ongoing military, political, economic, social, and ideological assault necessary to secure this land. The historical and current conditions for Palestinians, involving nearly 70 years of systematic ethnic cleansing and apartheid control in the name of political Zionism, thus pose an enormous moral challenge.

The list of human rights abuses perpetrated by the government of Israel in its present occupation of Palestine forms a catalogue of terror: the killing and breaking the bones of defenseless demonstrators, arming Israeli settlers to commit acts of violence against

Palestinians, bombing of hospitals and schools, home incursion and demolition, the use of toxic gas, mass arrests, detention, and torture—including the torture of children. It is estimated that since 1967, one third of all Palestinian men have been held in detention by Israeli forces, often without charges being brought against them and not infrequently for decades. Almost all of such detainees are mistreated and torture is so common that the physical and psychological consequences of torture by the Israelis form an important public health problem in Palestine. More insidious forms of community reprisal imposed by the Israelis involve the deliberate, systematic, and massive destruction of the economic, agricultural, educational, and legal systems in Palestine as well as the maintenance of total control over its roadways, water, air space, human movement, and natural resources. The deliberate effort to decimate the leadership of Palestinian society through specific targeting of Palestinian journalists, attorneys, human rights advocates, community organizers, and legislators—including prominent mental health professionals and their families—has been an especially malignant aspect of Israeli policy.

The violent displacement, containment, and devastation of the people of Palestine could never have been achieved without the astronomical and ever-increasing quantity of military support given to the government of Israel by the United States—more cumulative military aid since the end of World War II than to any other country, estimated to be nearly $100 billion dollars—motivated by its own geopolitical interests in the Middle East. And this war of tanks and fighter jets has been justified through a war of words, a well-financed propaganda campaign that portrays the Israelis as brave victims defending democracy and the Palestinians as dehumanized dangerous fanatics.

The distortions of fact undergirding pro-Israeli propaganda and the details of Israeli crimes against humanity have been documented by tireless reportage by the United Nations, by human rights organizations such as Amnesty International, and international organizations against torture, and by international scholars and journalists; an increasingly vocal number of Israeli organizations and courageous individuals in Israel speak out against the oppression of the Palestinian people by their own government and its pernicious effects on Israeli society as well as Palestinian society. Movements to educate and persuade the global public in solidarity with the Palestinian community have emerged in many places, dedicated to exposing the violent aggression, racism, and violation of international standards of human rights perpetrated by the state of Israel.

The role of mental health workers

Mental health professionals, skilled by training and experience to listen to agendas hidden beneath the surface, have the potential to defuse the power of the pro-Israeli propaganda narrative through distinguishing fantasy from fact and through identifying the motivating denial, self-interest, and self-deception behind its assertions. One such propaganda position, fundamental to the worldview of political Zionism, asserts the inherent "specialness" of the Jewish people: special in their history of victimization in Europe, the Jewish people require an ethnocentric militarized state that is beyond criticism and exempt from international law. While playing on the guilt of the West for its passivity and collaboration with the Holocaust of World War II, the questionable assertion of Israeli specialness presents a seemingly innocent surface while obliterating moral accountability for the covert colonialist greed, entitlement, and ruthless violence of the Israeli government by equating all criticism with anti-Semitism.

Another propaganda position is the oft-heard "liberal" view that Israeli violence—although lamentable—is mirrored and justified by the threat of Palestinian violence; the questionable assertion of symmetry presents a surface of tragic inevitability with an apparently even-handed dispersal of blame and empathy on both sides, while covertly normalizing and supporting the status quo. And overall, the mental health professional will recognize in the Israeli mistreatment of the Palestinian people the contours characteristic of abuse dynamics: the abuse itself and the ensuing relentless campaign to undermine the credibility of the victim, to destroy the victim's self-respect, and to delegitimize and silence the victim's narrative. By identifying propaganda manipulations such as these as politically motivated distortions, rather than self-evident truths, mental health professionals can elevate the level of reality-testing within discussion of Israel and occupied Palestine.

In addition to bringing insight to discourse on the occupation, the mental health community is in a unique position to properly assess the gravity of the immense psychological and social damage being inflicted by the occupation through a professional understanding of the emotional consequences of war, occupation, and pervasive insecurity, and especially through the viewpoint of child development. Through these lenses, the overt atrocities that now achieve public prominence in viral internet video clips (such as Israeli soldiers beating a Palestinian child) can be placed in a larger context of overall violence, racism, social fragmentation, detention without due process, unemployment, impoverishment, malnutrition, family dysfunction, humiliation, and human misery and the devastating everyday impact of all of these factors on psychological well-being. The psychological assault of 1948 was simple—designed to instill fear with the goal of inducing Palestinians to abandon their homes; but the psychological assault of today is sophisticated—designed to destroy Palestinian morale, to induce a state of passive hopelessness, and to undermine the sources of individual, family, and social cohesion. The goal today is to achieve the pervasive psychological isolation and surrender in an entire captive population which has nowhere to go and to crush Palestinian resistance at its roots in the human spirit.

The effects of the occupation on all sectors of Palestinian society is thus the driving force for a major burden of mental health distress afflicting millions of individuals, a distress in which very high rates of common psychiatric disorders such as depression, anxiety, and post-traumatic stress disorder have been documented. But unlike the damage to a community in the wake of an earthquake or a flood, the harm to the Palestinian people includes and exceeds the domain of acute injury; the Palestinian people have suffered from chronic injury inflicted by chronic injustice. Under occupation, the people of Palestine face a purposefully inflicted degradation of the entire system of meaning which has given them identity as a people. Not only individual selves but the collective self has been damaged. We are challenged as healers to think in new ways to develop comprehensive theories and practices appropriate to this context.

In our view, the mental health community is especially equipped to be active and proactive in addressing these clinical and—at the same time—moral challenges both in our daily practice whenever these issues arise and beyond, through our professional organizations and activities. Our professional skills as active listeners, as clarifiers of contradictions, as confronters of confused thought, as persuaders in the community and care-givers to the suffering, and as defenders of justice for the vulnerable and the victimized—these skills prepare mental health workers to be useful in multiple ways in the struggle against the occupation.

We encourage mental health workers first to do no harm: for example, to speak out against the participation of fellow professionals in roles which advance the practices of the occupation, such as assisting in the development of "interrogation" techniques. In addition, we encourage mental health workers to join projects to open the scope of debate, to witness, to document, and to engage in research addressing the occupation and to seek out partnerships with Palestinians to expose the full extent of its consequences. There is great need to support Palestinian initiatives that provide direct mental health services for patients and foster forms of community life which are genuinely therapeutic for the Palestinian public. As mental health workers, we have skills as clinicians and trainers which may be of practical use on the ground.

But just as no mental health professional would treat a victim of ongoing incest or torture without "calling the authorities," no mental health professional can treat a victim of occupation in a vacuum. Our duty to report abuse is part of our professionalism and in many instances is codified in statute as our legal obligation. The abuse must stop or all of our therapeutic efforts will be meaningless or perhaps even harmful, because victims of abuse need justice in the world as well as therapy. The treatment of victims of violence is thus multi-disciplinary in its essence, because outside forces such as the police and the court systems are required to restore fundamental rights to the injured parties, acting in coordination with mental health as a discipline. It is consistent with our mandate as healers that we integrate public health agendas that examine and take action to address the root causes of human suffering. Therefore human rights must matter to mental health workers, requiring activism in response to their violation and disregard.

The psychological and psychiatric consequences of the Israeli occupation are not only mental health events but legal and geopolitical events; restoring mental well-being requires us to call for the intervention of moral and legal authorities with international stature. Just as professional organizations in mental health have cooperated with legislators and judges to create and to enforce laws protecting the victims of incest, rape, and family violence, thus too the mental health community must work in mutually supportive ways with legal, political, and human rights organizations to seek justice for the Palestinian people and restoration of its human dignity.

Thus, as concerned professionals, we may need to move beyond the confines of our accustomed professional roles and to act as a group in support of movements to achieve a genuine transformation in Israel and in occupied Palestine that respects the human needs and human rights of all who live there. We must commit ourselves not only to work as clinicians for the liberation of the individual but for the liberation of the community. We call upon mental health professionals to engage in sociopolitical solidarity with the people of Palestine as a therapeutic position. Dedicating ourselves to this work while the occupation continues will give us the insights we will need in the future, as facilitators involved in the process of reconciliation. Laying down a foundation of involvement during a time of crisis prepares us for participating in a resolution to the crisis that will bring genuine redress, justice, and full civil rights to the people of Palestine.

Global Solidarity With Palestinians: From psychological support to political change

Originally published in *Middle East Monitor*, 30 December 2014

As the hundreds of thousands of people around the world who protested the massacres in Gaza retreat into inertia, hypnotized by news about the ceasefire and the Gaza reconstruction conference, a more insidious process of Israeli land confiscations, settlement expansion and control over Jerusalem's holy places continues to erode Palestinian life. Lynch mobs of young Jewish Israelis continue to organize themselves in preparation for another attack on Palestinians, and the Israeli military enjoys impunity for its war crimes in Gaza. To Palestinians, the ceasefire means a return to being the blind spot of the world's conscience—a less dramatic assault on life's freedoms, with its daily humiliations and oppression.

The parroting by world leaders of "Israel's right to self-defense" causes further injury to Palestinians, given all the hostility and violence inflicted on us. It's no wonder that Palestinians experience the outside world as biased, selfish and complicit in harming us. Indeed, just as a rape victim feels doubly traumatized by the indifference of the bystander, Palestinians feel betrayed by the world's silence. Like the rape victim, Palestinians need and deserve not only the sympathy of the individual but the delivery of justice.

But thanks to all those who demonstrate on our behalf, recognizing us and validating our experience, letting us know that we are seen and heard, our belief in the fairness and goodness of others is not completely destroyed.

International solidarity with the Palestinians helps assuage the psychological pain and alienation caused by Israel's relentless dehumanization and the world's apathy, denial and denunciation. Local and international initiatives that help Palestinians survive, recover, attain their freedom and sustain their struggle facilitate engagement and restore a sense of health to Palestinian society and protect against despair and extremism. Palestinians are, in fact, fond of internationals; it is never in Palestine that internationals are kidnapped and beheaded!

While demonstrations provide Palestinians important psychological support, and an opportunity for demonstrators to vent their objections and frustrations, they so far have failed to change our political reality or prevent a future massacre against us. Israel does not respond to moral condemnation, and Washington's support for Israel goes beyond political statements to financing Israeli military aggression with Americans' tax dollars.

In the face of our political leaders' deafness, solidarity activists must work to gain momentum and adopt innovative strategies and tools. This will require a global as well as regional grassroots commitment to the well-being of the Palestinian people, involving active and long-term mobilization of ideological, judicial, political and economic solidarity.

It is imperative to build on the instinctive, immediate, reflexive feelings of empathy and solidarity to achieve a more long-term, sober and strategic globalized solidarity movement that can act as a unified entity governed by mutual cooperation. Such an entity can create alliances and coalitions among different groups, and orchestrate, multiply and augment the impact of the solidarity movement. Not only can it serve as an umbrella to many individual sympathizers—Arabs, Israelis, Germans—who, intimidated in their own societies, are unable to establish solidarity organizations there, but it can protect them and facilitate communication between them and their own governments.

Global solidarity requires a horizontal (preaching to the non-converted) as well as vertical (creating access to power) network of associations. While the former aims to achieve an improved level of literacy regarding Palestine in the face of an international public intoxicated by Israeli propaganda, the latter requires formal training on advocacy strategies (e.g., media campaigns, public speaking, lobbying and social media) of a smaller group focused on legislation and other institutional decisions.

Solidarity with Palestinians means uniting and binding together, based not on family, religion, ethnicity or class, but on shared values and a common goal of liberating Palestine from occupation, restoring justice and human rights to Palestinians, and holding Israel accountable to international law. Solidarity requires learning to work in spite of and through our divisions, as well as the commitment of people who don't share our pain or life conditions but refuse to be either passive or active collaborators in our oppression—people who view the liberation of Palestine as integral to their own self-liberation.

I have met many of these passionate, sincere people, and am convinced that learning how to effect political change will protect many of them from burnout. There is no single recipe for solidarity—as the French say, *"Chacun fait sa cuisine interne,"* (everyone creates his own worldview)—so just as I ask people in solidarity to let Palestinians choose their means of resistance, it is important to respect the choices of the means of solidarity of the citizens of each county: they know best what works for them. It is important, nevertheless, to be flexible and open to consultation and collaboration with others.

Basic to the establishment of a global solidarity movement is encouraging partnership and teamwork with Palestinian professionals, academics, activists and educators, so that solidarity actions are sensitive to the needs and culture of Palestinian civil society, and helping Palestinians to disseminate their narrative, aspirations and point of view to a wider world.

Crisis as opportunity

Palestinian national cohesion is the prerequisite for global solidarity. The partition of Palestine's political parties that occurred in the wake of our 2006 elections, and which has been exacerbated by external political and financial aid provided to some Palestinians and not others, caused significant damage to Palestinian morale and values, and has likewise fragmented solidarity efforts with Palestinians.

But the brutality of Israel's latest attack on Gaza created a spontaneous, passionate and popular feeling of national unity, which the Palestinian leadership had no option but to join. This, therefore, is an opportunity for Palestinians to build on their rejection of polarization, incitement and intimidation, and to invest in the vigor and vitality and mobilization of energies and achievements in various spheres of life. The steadfastness of our compatriots in Gaza elevated the morale of the people and improved levels of social cohesion and trust. Trust in turn generates teamwork and mutual cooperation, and increases the level of national identity and the desire to participate in public life.

During Israel's assault on Gaza, Palestinians did not identify with the positions of our (long-ago) elected leaders, but with the resistance. As a result, the majority of Palestinians now challenge the Palestinian Authority, reject its coordination of security with Israel, and demand it take our case to the International Court of Justice. For this energetic response to continue, to be more than just a temporary reaction. It is crucial to support the growth of fully responsible democratic institutions within Palestine that will coordinate governing and self-sustaining economic structures in a wise, efficient and responsive manner. Adherence to the principles of meritocracy, transparency and accountability is a prerequisite for establishing institutional reform and participatory citizenship; developing a Palestinian national charter, with the participation of all political parties, to be placed before voters in a referendum, is also a mandatory step toward consolidating national unity.

Helping Palestinians and Israelis alike

In addition to promoting healing and creating political change, including preventing future attacks and furthering Palestinian liberation, solidarity with the Palestinians also will serve to diminish the thirst for revenge and pave the way for future reconciliation. Because it facilitates both personal revival and social reform, it eventually will help Palestinians and Israelis alike in a post-war era that we hope will come soon. The safety in which it envelops us promotes trust and allows for mutual acknowledgement and compassion, thereby paving the way for forgiveness and justice—the foundation of peace.

The ICJ Hearing On Genocide Contributes To Healing Palestinian Historical Trauma

Originally published on *Middle East Monitor*, 19 January 2024

Israel's appearance before the International Court of Justice (ICJ) at the Hague is an important step on the road to justice and a necessary contribution to the healing of the historical trauma of the Palestinian people. This trauma began with the Balfour Declaration of 1917 and has continued through the Nakba of 1948, and through many subsequent wars and aggressions. The trauma is present in the genocide we are living now, which is deepening and expanding our historical wounds to a point that cannot heal without a profound intervention.

The state of Israel has always transgressed international law. The powers of Europe and the United States have colluded with it. The United Nations has failed to deter it or hold it accountable for its violations. The Palestinians have always been acutely aware of this injustice and abandonment, of betrayal after betrayal. Israel's impunity throughout history has enforced a sense of isolation for the Palestinians and has weakened our faith in human interconnection and fairness.

South Africa's actions at the ICJ—regardless of their results—came to correct, at least partially, that flaw in the Palestinian perspective of the world, through its solidarity, recognition and support.

The appearance of Israel at the ICJ conveys significant symbolism for our humanitarian cause. South Africa, the main engine driving the trial, is an icon of confrontation and triumph over racial and ethnic oppression. Its arguments holding Israel accountable for the charge of genocide supports the rights of Palestinians and confronts Western powers and their system of international subjugation with their complicity in an ethnic tyranny that has stained their hands with blood.

We welcome the people of Africa, the victims of past violations of human rights, in solidarity with the Palestinians—the victims of the present. This solidarity liberates us from the humiliation born from our exclusion from the conscience of the human community. It promises us that there is still goodness in the world. It gives us confidence in our shared humanity. It lights a glimmer of hope that there is fairness and justice in a world that has darkened our lives with oppression for over a century.

Most of us in Palestine believe in a heavenly court and in divine justice. All the same, we recognize that religious faith should not be an obstacle to the relentless pursuit of justice here on earth. The great importance of international trials lies in giving voice to those who have been victimized by injustice. This action repairs psychological injury and renders us effective survivors; it fortifies us in bringing those responsible for crimes to make proper reparation, so that their crimes do not pass without just condemnation. Calling those responsible to account is crucial as a deterrent for them and for all others.

This week, Egyptians took to the streets chanting, "They did it, Mandela's grandchildren, while we are in fear, shame and humiliation." Perhaps that was their reaction to the Israeli defence team's claims that Egypt is responsible for closing the border to Gaza and preventing the delivery of aid. Namibia added its voice to that of

South Africa, maybe in reaction to Germany, who had joined in the court process to support Israel, as if encouraging the current extermination of Palestinians could atone for the German history of exterminating the Jewish people along with many others. Namibia reminded the court of the German crimes against the people of Namibia, helping reveal the full history of the current actors at the Hague.

South Africa's solidarity with Palestine gives us hope for the global movement resisting racial discrimination. Palestinians and their supporters must take full advantage of this historic moment. We must continue to work within a variety of frameworks and by all avenues, whether through professional organizations, trade unions, diplomatic channels, or the pressure of street demonstrations. We must affirm the rights of Palestinians, make a record of their sufferings and confront their oppressors.

This mission will require concerted efforts, steadfastness in facing our challenges and extraordinary patience. Even if the road is long, the trial at the Hague and these advocacy measures can be a catalyst for genuine peace based on justice and on re-establishing Palestine's long-violated rights. This is an inspiring moment to activate a strong international movement which calls for the end of the historic occupation of Palestine, to set right this injustice and to highlight the untold harms Palestinians have endured for so many decades. Our duty now is to hold fast and to spare no effort at both the popular and the political levels—to bring into being a global renewal spearheaded by the courage of this historic moment at the International Court of Justice.

'A World Without Borders': Revolutionary love and solidarity for Palestine

Originally published on *Middle East Monitor*, 16 July 2024

A World Without Borders, read the tattoo on the arm of one of the Brazilian activists who stood with me and my Palestinian friend at the São Paulo airport, bidding us farewell before our return flight. When unexpected challenges arose, the Brazilian activists stayed with us for hours, helping to resolve the issues. Even when we were denied access to our flight that night, they insured that we had a place to sleep and continued to handle the logistics while we rested. This affectionate support exemplifies the solidarity I encounter around the world. For someone transitioning from the hostility of the occupied land, such experiences are like an emotional thermal shock.

A world without borders, racism, and political violence is a collective dream, connecting stateless Palestinians with many people worldwide in what can be called revolutionary love—a love that is not declared, but deeply felt in the hands that connect, the hearts that heal, and the minds that envision a world where freedom and equality are inherent rights for all.

Revolutionary love manifests in small, everyday actions: the teacher in a refugee camp providing hope to children who have known only violence; the artist who tells stories of the resilience of a forgotten people; the ordinary citizens boycotting products that contribute to oppression and supporting fair trade and ethical businesses. Each of these actions contributes to a larger movement of solidarity and liberation.

Revolutionary love is not just an abstract concept. It is a transformative force that challenges the status quo and fuels the fight for justice, equality, and human dignity. It is the courage to love beyond visible and invisible boundaries, to empathize with those whose suffering is often silenced and normalized, and to act in solidarity with their struggles. It is the energy that allows us to stand up and make sacrifices for one another.

Remember the story of Rachel Corrie, an American activist who stood in front of Israeli bulldozers to protect Palestinian homes from demolition? Her ultimate sacrifice of life itself exemplifies revolutionary love, demonstrating a willingness to face immense personal risk for the sake of justice. Or think of the countless medical professionals from around the world who volunteer in Gaza, providing critical healthcare amid bombings and blockades. Their acts of service, driven by deep empathy and commitment to human dignity, transcend national, religious, ethnic and cultural divides. Watch students facing police violence in campus encampments in North America and Europe. Read about Zionist groups like Canary Mission and pro-Israel leagues threatening people's jobs and jeopardizing their institutional standing for speaking up for Palestinians.

Unlike paid missionaries who join the Israeli army's genocidal war in Gaza for a few thousand euros per week, and the bribed journalists and influencers who spread anti-Palestinian propaganda, we see activists who stand beside Palestinians. They raise their voices in tireless advocacy against genocide. They offer daily support to those who refuse to succumb to despair despite relentless adversity. They receive no money for these principled acts and indeed often must pay a price themselves for their commitment, through suffering tangible and intangible and tangible losses.

The call for international solidarity with the Palestinian people is rooted in revolutionary love. It is reciprocal, even when Palestinians' hands are tied and we cannot extend them to our comrades in equal measure. For decades, Palestinians have been immersed in personal and collective hardships, our lives subject to relentless scrutiny and control. Yet, amid this darkness, the feeling that we are connected to a wider human community has not perished. I remember Palestinian public employees contributing a small percentage of their salary to Syrian refugees on several occasions. Similarly, Palestinians demonstrated in solidarity with the Turkish people who lost their lives protecting their democracy in 2016 and demonstrated in support of the oppressed Rohingya people in Burma. In Gaza, I witnessed people collecting money to support the survivors of earthquakes in Turkey and Syria as well as the victims of flooding in Libya. Palestinian health and mental health professionals as well have participated in support missions to several crisis areas worldwide. It is a testament to the strength of revolutionary love that Palestinians continue to strive for connections with indigenous, Black, and other marginalized communities.

I believe that human beings have an innate need for justice and empathy. This is my understanding of "*fitrah*," translated as "original disposition," in Islamic faith. When we witness suffering, our capacity for empathy compels us to act. This is not merely a moral obligation but a psychological imperative that connects us to our shared humanity. Revolutionary love taps into this deep-seated need, urging us to break down the learned barriers of indifference and prejudice that often divide us.

Supporting the Palestinian struggle is about recognizing and affirming the humanity of a people who have been dehumanized for far too long. We Palestinians find ourselves at the climax of a clash of civilizations, challenging not only Israel, but a unipolar and deformed world order, where human dignity and rights are divided unevenly. This deformed world presents us with ambiguous and illusionary borders between Occident and Orient, the global North and the global South. In this corrupt world order, the Israeli occupation sitting on our chests is considered to be very European, Western, and civilized while we are viewed as barbaric and dehumanized savages.

Palestinians dare to push Israel off our chests and in doing so challenge White supremacy and the Western world order. We should not be alone is doing so. A world that claims to regret Black slavery and the eradication of the indigenous people in the conquest of new continents should be in solidarity with Palestinians. Revolutionary love means seeing your ancestors in our eyes, hearing their voices in our cries. Revolutionary love is about understanding that Palestinian pain is universal and that our dreams are legitimate and human. It is about acknowledging our right to push away the heavy weight on our chest, to breathe and to connect as equals.

International solidarity with the Palestinian people means amplifying our voices, supporting our rights, and standing with us in our defense of our common human dignity. As the poet Samih Choukeir puts it: "If my voice fades, your throats will not," emphasizing that the collective spirit of solidarity will continue unabated in the struggle for justice. It means educating oneself and others in Palestinian history and current realities. Possessing this knowledge makes plain the similarity between our struggle and that of other native and colonized nations. This knowledge prepares us for challenging harmful narratives and advocating for global political change to promotes human rights for all.

By embracing revolutionary love, we affirm that the struggle to end the occupation of Palestine is a struggle driven by love for humanity, not hate—contrary to what our enemies falsely claim. It is a call to action, urging people of the world to stand together, not as passive bystanders but as active participants in the fight for justice. In doing so, we not only honor the Sumud and the courage of the Palestinian people, but also uphold the values that define our shared human experience: compassion, justice, and unwavering love.

In supporting the Palestinian people, you not only aid our struggle, you enrich your own lives by connecting with a deeper sense of purpose and humanity. Revolutionary love teaches us that our fates are intertwined, that justice for one is justice for all. A world without borders—let us answer this call with open hearts and determined spirits, standing together in defense of human dignity and enduring peace.

Epilogue

Radiance In Pain And Resilience: The global reverberation of Palestinian historical trauma

This transcript of the Edward Said Lecture, presented by Dr Samah Jabr on 20 February 2024, was published on Princeton University website, 27 February 2024

Ladies and gentlemen, esteemed guests—I stand before you today with deep reverence and a sense of purpose as we gather for the Edward Said Memorial Lecture. At this moment, Palestine is going through one of the most difficult confrontations it has ever endured. What Said might have said about this confrontation is a question that crosses many of our minds. We are not here to second-guess what he might have observed, yet we can draw inspiration from his intellectual legacy—a heritage that sheds light on our dark reality and helps us to see the path forward out of its obscurity.

When I think of Said's absence at this time, I'm reminded of the words of the Abbasi poet knight Abu Firas AlHamadani, prisoner in the Byzantine capital of Constantinople: "My people will mention me when the matter is serious; in the dark night the full moon is indispensable."

Respected audience—our exploration, entitled Radiance in Pain and Resilience: The Global Reverberation of Palestinian Historical Trauma, is an invitation to embark on a journey into the complex web of cultural identity, psychological resilience, and enduring wounds that is manifest in our history. The Palestinian narrative is one fraught with displacement, dispossession, and cultural distortion interwoven with threads of struggle and resilience.

Edward Said, himself a Palestinian exile, exemplified the fusion of intellectual rigor with a passionate commitment to justice. His life and work guide us to confront uncomfortable truths and to navigate the profound psychological dimensions of our history. His insights have shaped my understanding of the complexities inherent in the Palestinian experience; his vision has encouraged me to question the validity of many of the dominant Western concepts and language in psychiatry, and to assess their applicability to the Palestinian context.

Ladies and gentlemen—it was before October 7th when I accepted the kind invitation to speak before you; but the subsequent military attacks on Gaza serve as brutal reminders of the long ongoing struggle faced by the Palestinian people. The relentless violence of this moment perpetuates a state of protracted distress, amplifying the trauma embedded in the historical narrative. To comprehend the depth of this trauma, we must delve into the psychological repercussions on the individual and the collective psyche, and understand the interplay between historical wounds and the Palestinian quest for well-being and liberation.

In the midst of displacement, where homes become dust and landscapes are transformed into pale shadows of an inaccessible past, the psychological toll on both individuals and communities is immeasurable. The assessment unit focused on an individual human being alone does not tell the whole story. The enduring impact of historical trauma is found not only in physical dislocation but also in dislocation within the intricate architecture of the mind and the relational webs of the community. Historical and current trauma influence the capacity for representation, and for social and psychological well-being. It is within this context that we find ourselves compelled to explore the multifaceted dimensions of Palestinian history and mental health.

Palestinian historical trauma

Respected colleagues—individual trauma theory and the popular diagnosis of PTSD fail to fully capture the Palestinians' experience of historical trauma—a deliberate trauma which has no clear beginning or end. The symptoms of historical trauma are not limited to re-experiencing, hyperarousal and avoidance. Trauma in Palestine is colonial, continuous, collective, cumulative and cross-generational; it reverberates into every domain of Palestinian life, health, identity, culture and economy.

The ancient and multicultural capital of Jerusalem has been transformed into a Jewish city; this and the imposition of Israeli curricula on Palestinian schoolchildren, the fragmentation of families across checkpoints, the constriction of human movement imposed by identity papers, and the erasure of Palestinian culture, history and language cannot be measured by a PTSD checklist. Demolishing Palestinian homes, burning their olive groves, imposing nudity on Palestinians, forcing them to kiss the Israeli flag or to dance to the Israeli national anthem in exchange for basic needs are not considered traumatic events according to psychiatry books. Historical trauma theory suggests that lives are lived in specific historical times and places. As the scholar Glen elder has observed, "If historical times and places change, they change the way people live their lives." (2001)

Here are four assumptions underlying historical trauma theory:

(1) Mass trauma is deliberately and systematically inflicted upon a target population by a subjugating, dominant population.

(2) Trauma is not limited to a single catastrophic event, but continues over an extended period of time.

(3)   Traumatic events reverberate throughout the population, creating a widespread experience of trauma.

(4)   The magnitude of the trauma experience derails the population from its natural developmental course—resulting in a legacy of physical, psychological, social, and economic discontinuities that are transmitted intergenerationally and persist.

Colleagues, in Palestine, the political is very personal and very psychological. As I wrote these words, I heard in my mind the cries of 15-year-old Palestinian girl Layan Hamadeh, who was fatally shot in her family automobile while calling the Palestine Red Crescent society team for help. Layan had been trapped within the vehicle after an ambush, along with the bodies of members of her family. We could hear the shooting and her cries, which grew louder and louder and then disappeared.

Layan's six-year-old sister, Hind, also trapped in the car, had survived for several hours as the Red Crescent team attempted to rescue her—but 12 days later, Hind and the rescue team were found dead.

As I wrote this story, I received a news report from the north of the Gaza Strip where the bodies of 30 Gazans were discovered handcuffed behind their back, blindfolded, and executed; their corpses were then covered with trash and rubble. We can imagine the psychological effects of such events on those who knew those people and loved them, their family members, colleagues, neighbors, classmates.

Such events are capable of traumatizing anyone who has heard of them. They awaken vivid memories of an endless number of similar accounts stretching across the past century; from Deir Yasine, to Tantoura and Kufor Qasem to Jenin, everywhere and everytime Israel has killed Palestinians on their native land.

Colleagues, the occupation, as part of its necro-politics, has deliberately targeted the health system, the major lifeline of Palestinians. It has thus created in Gaza deadly conditions which are now self-sustaining, even if a ceasefire were to be enforced today.

A population of 1.8 million displaced, malnourished people have been concentrated in Rafah during winter; pandemic respiratory infections and hepatitis are rampant, and people are dying of their untreated infected wounds as famine is looming in Gaza. By early February, 340 medical personnel have been killed, 125 ambulances destroyed, 26 out of the 36 Gazan hospitals have been demolished, the rest are rendered partially dysfunctional, 100 doctors have been arrested and exposed to torture; the details of the torture of Dr Mohammad AlRen and Dr Muhammad Abu Silmeyeh are chilling. Torture of arrested doctors is used to extract false testimonies before cameras; such statements are then utilized to support the Israeli claim that the Palestinian resistance has used hospitals as bunkers. Torture is used to destroy these physicians psychologically and break their image as role models of post-traumatic growth for all they have given during this crisis, and to intimidate their colleagues into abandoning their commitment to serve their people. Chilling also is the official international media and institutional silence about this unprecedented attack on Gaza and its health system in particular.

Denial
Now let me talk to you about denial. We cannot treat something if we do not acknowledge its existence. Denial and suppression of

awareness of the historical trauma of Palestine impedes its treatment. In the documentary film *1948: Creation and Catastrophe*, the Israeli historian Ilan Pappe explains the fate of Arab villages. In 1947, there were 500 to 700 of these villages in the land that eventually became Israel. By the end of 1948, only about 100 of those village remained. Pape explains how Israel planted forests of pine trees on the resulting debris, to erase the Arab character of these places and to obliterate their memory. Palestinians call this greenwashing ethnic cleansing. Then colonies were built with Hebrew names that resembled the original Arab names, in order to suggest that these were originally Jewish places. Rosemary Sayegh has written about the exclusion of the Palestinian Nakba from the "Trauma Genre" and examined crucial ways in which ignorance of Palestine and the Nakba of 1948 has been cultivated, whether through colonial appropriation, landscape transformation, censorship, memoricide, schooling, or promoting the fear of being labeled anti-Semitic.

Denial of the Palestinian historical trauma is also vivid in the discourse of the US government; in its repetition of the Israeli falsehoods of decapitated babies and weaponized rape. We see this denial in the statement of the American Psychiatric Association standing in solidarity with Israel, a statement that ignores a century of Palestinian political oppression. We see this denial in the threat of being labeled anti-Semitic, a specter which haunts American college campuses to silence students and academics alike and to threaten their future careers. We see this denial in an incitement of pervasive hostility towards Palestinians that has led to hate crimes, such as the fatal stabbing of the young boy Wadea al Fayoume and the unprovoked shooting of three Palestinian university students at Vermont, and in pointing a pistol towards Aaron Bushnel, the US airforce soldier who set himself on fire outside the Israeli embassy in Washington, DC, in an apparent act of protest against Israel's devastating war on Gaza and American complicity in it.

In the face of this overwhelming denial, everyone in Palestine realizes that this genocidal political violence is waged against us by Israel and its colonial supporters in the West, and that this assault is enabled by the United States's military, economy, media, politics and vetoes. The complicity of the United States is even known to Palestinian children who handle their own immense grief with temporary denial. One boy told his friend, "Your father was killed." The friend responded, "No, he's just sleeping; he's too tired." A girl asked a doctor who dressed her wounds: "Doctor, is this a dream or reality?" Another girl with an amputated foot inquired, "When will my foot grow back?" In time, these children recover from their denial and chant: "We will triumph; we will triumph against Israel and the United States," while the United States remains in denial for its responsibility in shedding Palestinian blood.

Treatment

Esteemed audience, at this moment, 6% of Gazans have been physically exterminated, wounded, or maimed. Everyone in Gaza is psychologically affected, and most Palestinians are experiencing anticipatory trauma, watching from afar in dread, survivor guilt, and helplessness. And because Palestine is an Arab, Muslim, and human cause, the radiance of our pain is so intense and vast. Some of you are suffering from trauma by proxy; the genocide has stirred up the traumatic history of natives, Blacks and people from the global South. But, bear in mind, this is not the only feeling that is radiating from Gaza.

Have you seen the heroic doctor Amira AlAssouli at Al-Nasr hospital taking off her jacket, crouching down, and running in front of snipers to rescue a young man? Did you watch the teenage Sir Isaac Newton of Gaza creating an electrical system to light up the tents of displaced people? Did you know the Al Jazeera correspondent, Wael AlDahdouh, overcame his personal grief over the death of his family members to continue his professional mission to expose the obliterated truth of what's going on in Gaza? The images of resilience and post-traumatic growth emerging from the rubble of Gaza are endless; people's virtues unfold as a force that enables individuals and communities to withstand the weight of historical trauma. It is in cultural expressions, communal bonds, and international solidarity that we witness the strong spirit of a people determined to express their love, to maintain prosocial action, and to reclaim their identity and agency—these are manifestations of the Palestinian notion of Sumud. From the poetry that echoes through refugee camps to the preservation of traditional arts and crafts, Palestinian culture becomes a testament to fortitude found in the face of adversity.

International solidarity, too, plays a pivotal role in the landscape of resilience. The global reverberation of Palestinian historical trauma transcends geographical boundaries, compelling individuals and communities worldwide to stand in solidarity with the Palestinian cause. It is through this interconnectedness that the radiance of resilience gains momentum, fostering a shared commitment to justice and human dignity.

The recent appearance of Israel before the International Court of Justice (ICJ) at The Hague is a crucial step towards justice and healing for the historical trauma endured by the Palestinian people. Israel's impunity and the lack of accountability have contributed to the isolation of Palestinians and has weakened their belief in global fairness. South Africa's actions at the ICJ, regardless of the outcome, have been perceived as a corrective measure, symbolically challenging ethnic tyranny and Western complicity in oppression.

The solidarity shown by Africa, a region with its own history of trauma and human rights violations, with the cause of Palestine instills hope in a shared humanity. Recent global reactions, such as Namibia highlighting German colonial crimes and its current hypocrisy in supporting Israel's attacks on Gaza, underscore the significance of the ICJ trial. This kind of solidarity is seen as an inspiration for a global movement against colonial powers and racial discrimination.

Palestinians and their supporters are urged to seize this historic moment, working through a multitude of channels to affirm rights, document sufferings, and confront oppressors. Genuine peace is rooted in justice and the current moment is viewed as an opportunity to activate a strong international movement, popular and political, spearheaded by the courage displayed at the International Court of Justice.

In conclusion, today's gathering is an invitation to engage in a nuanced understanding of the complexities surrounding historical trauma, to foster empathy, and to cultivate a space for healing and solidarity.

Edward Said's vision of intellectual responsibility serves as a guiding framework, challenging us to not only bear witness to the pain of others but to actively engage in the reconstruction of a more just world. It guides us to question dominant narratives, confront systemic injustices, and advocate for the rights of the opressed. In the face of historical trauma, intellectual responsibility becomes a compass—a call to action that transcends the confines of academia and permeates the realms of social and political change.

May the echoes of our collective reflections resonate beyond this lecture hall, contributing to the ongoing legacy of Edward Said's intellectual courage and compassion. Let us illuminate the path towards a future where historical trauma is not a shackle but a catalyst for positive change—a future where the radiance of resilience and solidarity prevails over the shadows of the past and its pain.

Final Words

The Kites Of Hope: Little Gaza's message to Earth

Originally written 18 March 2024

In a realm beyond the mortal plane, a Little Gaza existed in Paradise, a tranquil oasis untouched by the turmoil that had plagued its earthly counterpart. Here, amid the golden glow of eternal sunshine and the gentle rustle of palm trees, the souls of those who had perished in the brutal genocide found solace and sanctuary.

Among the inhabitants of Little Gaza were a myriad of souls—innocent children whose laughter had been silenced too soon, courageous freedom fighters who had dared to defy tyranny, resilient mothers and fathers who had shielded their loved ones from harm, brilliant university students whose dreams had been extinguished, dedicated journalists and doctors who had valiantly documented and treated the wounds of war, and the revered Palestinian thinkers and poets who had illuminated the path of resistance with their wisdom and insight.

Many of them had died under the rubble of their homes; some were executed in cold blood. A few were tortured to death, while others perished due to famine. Despite their diverse backgrounds, they were bound together by their shared struggle and steadfast spirit.

Amid their reveries, the souls of Little Gaza engaged in spirited discussions, reminiscing about their lives on Earth and sharing their hopes for the future of Palestine. They found solace in their collective memories and shared dreams, finding comfort in each other's company as they basked in the warmth of Paradise.

"I remember the sound of children's laughter," one soul murmured, a wistful smile playing across their ethereal features. "Even in the darkest of times, they found moments of joy."

"And the strength of the women," another soul added, their voice tinged with admiration. "They held their families together with a courage that knew no bounds."

The journalists among them spoke of the stories they had told, the truths they had uncovered, and the risks they had taken to shine a light on the plight of their people. "We may have fallen," one said sadly, "but our words live on, a testament to the power of truth." The doctors nodded in agreement, recalling the countless lives they had saved and the healing they had brought to a wounded land. "Our work may have been cut short," they said, "but our legacy endures in the hearts of those we cared for."

Their discussion was interrupted by the sound of fireworks. As they looked out from their heavenly space, the souls of Little Gaza bore witness to jubilant celebrations unfolding on Earth as Palestinians rejoiced in their hard-won national liberation. The disappearance of a military air force in the skies, the withdrawal of military tanks on the ground, the fall of the separation walls—the once frightening barriers of division and oppression—brought tears of joy to the eyes of the souls of Little Gaza. For years, they had yearned for this moment, dreaming of the day when their people would be free from the shackles of occupation.

As they watched the celebrations unfold far below, the souls of Little Gaza felt a sense of pride mingled with sorrow. Though they could no longer walk the streets of their city or feel the warmth of the sun on their skin, they knew that their spirits would forever be intertwined with the land they had called home.

Yet, even in their newfound Paradise, the souls of Little Gaza remained tethered to the plight of their people on Earth. They longed to reach out to their loved ones and comrades, to offer them solace and joy in their time of triumph. Inspired by the resilience of their earthly counterparts, they devised an arrangement to make their presence known to those still fighting for freedom.

With the poet Refaat Al Areer leading the way, the souls of Little Gaza crafted a brilliant plan to connect with their fellow Palestinians on Earth. They transformed the white cloth of their coffins, stained with the blood of their earthly struggles, into exquisite kites adorned with vibrant red poppies, symbolizing the resilience and beauty that had blossomed from their sacrifice. These magnificent kites soared through the heavens, carried in the air by gentle winds, weaving intricate patterns across the blue sky.

As the kites danced through outer space, the souls of Little Gaza watched with bated breath, their hearts filled with hope and longing. They knew that their message would reach their people on Earth, inspiring them to continue their fight for justice. And as they witnessed the tears of joy and determination in the eyes of their earthly comrades, they knew that their sacrifice had not been in vain.

On Earth, the people of Gaza looked up, astonished by the sight of the beautiful kites dancing in the sky. They felt a surge of emotion as they realized the significance of the message—a reminder of the sacrifices made for their freedom.

The kites, instead of drones, became a symbol of hope and resilience, inspiring the people of Gaza to continue their struggle for justice. In the days that followed, the people of Gaza welcomed home their refugees and celebrated the release of political detainees. Tears of joy flowed freely as families were reunited, and the streets echoed with songs of freedom and liberation.

As the echoes of Paradise reached their ears, the people of Gaza felt a renewed sense of determination. They knew that the spirits of Little Gaza were with them, guiding them on their path to a brighter future. And as they looked to the sky, they saw the kites soaring once more, a reminder that their dreams of freedom would never be forgotten. The souls of Little Gaza may have left behind the trials and tribulations of earthly existence, but their spirit lived on in the hearts of their people, inspiring them to continue their struggle until Palestine was truly free.

Wakefield Press is an independent publishing and
distribution company based in Adelaide, South Australia.
We love good stories and publish beautiful books.
To see our full range of books, please visit our website at
www.wakefieldpress.com.au
where all titles are available for purchase.
To keep up with our latest releases and news,
subscribe to the Wakefield Weekly at
https://mailchi.mp/wakefieldpress/subscribe

Find us!

Facebook: www.facebook.com/wakefield.press
Instagram: www.instagram.com/wakefieldpress

www.ingramcontent.com/pod-product-compliance
Lightning Source LLC
Chambersburg PA
CBHW040144270326
41929CB00024B/3368